Practical Manual on
Fish Nutrition and Feed Technology

The Authors

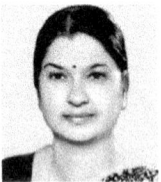

Dr. Priti Mishra is serving as 'Assistant Professor at the College of Fishery Science, Nanaji Deshmukh Veterinary Science University (NDVSU), Jabalpur, (M.P.). Prior to this, she had worked as 'Nutritionist' for about 14 years in the Phoenix Group, Jabalpur and has wide technical experience in Poultry, Livestock and Fish Nutrition. She has published two books chapters and more than '25 Research Papers/Popular Articles' in different Journals of National and International repute and presented many scientific papers on various conferences.

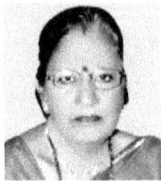

Dr. Neera Jain, M.Sc., Ph.D, formerly Associate Professor (Veterinary Biochemistry) in College of Veterinary Science and A.H., Nanaji Deshmukh Veterinary Science University (NDVSU), Jabalpur, (M.P.). She has the honor of receiving 'Prof. Nils Lagerl of Memorial Medal' by Indian Veterinary Association, Chennai for the best research paper in Indian Veterinary Journal (1995), publication of a review article in Animal Breeding Abstract, CAB International, England in 2003. Besides this she has authored 2 books and 40 research papers in National and International Journals of repute.

Practical Manual on
Fish Nutrition and Feed Technology

— Authors —

Priti Mishra

Assistant Professor
College of Fishery Science

Neera Jain

Associate Professor
Department of Veterinary Biochemistry
College of Veterinary Science & Animal Husbandry

Nanaji Deshmukh Veterinary Science University,
Jabalpur – 482 002, M.P.

2018

Daya Publishing House®

A Division of

Astral International Pvt. Ltd.
New Delhi – 110 002

Cataloging in Publication Data--DK
Courtesy: D.K. Agencies (P) Ltd. <docinfo@dkagencies.com>

Mishra, Priti, author.
Practical manual on fish nutrition and feed technology / authors, Priti Mishra, Neera Jain.
pages cm
ISBN 9789387057753 (International Edition)

1. Fishes--Nutrition. 2. Fishes--Feeding and feeds. I. Jain, Neera (Associate professor of veterinary biochemistry), author. II. Title. III. Title: Fish nutrition and feed technology.

LCC SH156.M57 2017 | DDC 639.3   23

Published by   : **Daya Publishing House®**
A Division of
Astral International Pvt. Ltd.
– ISO 9001:2015 Certified Company –
4736/23, Ansari Road, Darya Ganj
New Delhi-110 002
Ph. 011-43549197, 23278134
E-mail: info@astralint.com
Website: www.astralint.com

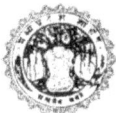

U.K. Purohit
Director

मत्स्योद्योग विभाग
FISHERIES DEPARTMENT
संचालनालय मत्स्योद्योग, मध्यप्रदेश
DIRECTORATE OF FISHERIES, MADHYA PRADESH
आधारतल विन्ध्याचल भवन, भोपाल - 462004
BASEMENT VINDHYACHAL BHAWAN, BHOPAL - 462004

Foreword

    I feel immense pleasure in writing the foreword for "*Practical Manual on Fish Nutrition and Feed Technology.*" This manual will be useful for B.F.Sc. Students. This is written as per syllabus prescribed by ICAR, New Delhi. The authors have covered all topics of course outline in details. The language is simple, thus easily understandable by students.

    I am sure that this manual will help students in understanding the basics of fish nutrition and feed technology to students of fisheries science at under graduate level.

22.7.15

U.K. Purohit
Director Fisheries
Madhya Pradesh

आधारतल विन्ध्याचल भवन, भोपाल - 462004
BASEMENT VINDHYACHAL BHAWAN, BHOPAL - 462004
☎ : 0755-2551542, Fax : 0755-2551357
Website : www.mpfisheries.nic.in, E-mail : dirfish@mp.nic.in

Preface

A comprehensive Manual is an unavoidable asset in the modern style of teaching. Since the introduction of all India syllabus by Indian Council of Agricultural Research (ICAR), the necessity to publish a Manual was felt. An attempt has been made to present this manual, keeping in view the needs of students offering courses in Fish Nutrition and Feed Technology at undergraduate level. The subject matter involves the matter from the books available for the purpose. The language is simple and easily understandable by the students.

Though the authors have tried to cover all topics in all possible required details, the suggestions for the improvement are cordially invited.

Priti Mishra
Neera Jain

Contents

Foreword   v

Preface   vii

1. General Precautions in Laboratory   1

2. Definition of Terms and Explanatory Notes   5

3. Indicators   9

4. Glasswares/Articles in Use and their Cleaning   11

5. General Precautions during Weighing   15

6. Preparation of Solutions and their Preservation   17

7. Proximate Principles in Feed: General View   23

8. Determination of Energy Value of Foods   41

9. Estimation of Salt Contents in Foods   45

10. Colorimetric Method of Estimation of Proteins   47

11. Colorimetric Method of Estimation of Carbohydrates   49

12. Paper Chromatography and Thin Layer Chromatography 51

13 Use of pH Meter 59

14. Estimation of β-Carotene 65

15. Preparation of Artificial Feeds 67

16. Determination of Sinking Rate and Stability of Feeds 73

17. Effect of Storage on Feed Quality 77

18. Estimation of Quality of Fish 87

19. Nutritional Requirement and Management of Supplementary
    Feeding in Cultured Freshwater Fish and Shellfish 95

    Appendix 101

1

General Precautions in Laboratory

The necessity for precautions arises while working in laboratory. The hazards are caused mainly by the chemicals and due to carelessness, untidiness and unsatisfactory working conditions. Therefore, following precautions are advocated:

General Precautions

1. Laboratory floor, working tables and water sinks should be kept neat and clean and it should be well ventilated and provided with an exhaust fan to remove unwanted gases, fumes and smoke.

2. One should work fully protected in laboratory by wearing white drill aprons and shoes.

3. Store chemicals and glassware in alphabetical order in well protected cupboards.

4. Always use acid and alkali gloves while handling strong acids and alkalies.

5. Distilled water bottles should be kept tightly corked to avoid absorption of atmospheric gases.

6. Dangerous chemicals include corrosive substances, volatile substances and organic solvents. Such chemicals should be handled carefully.

Handling of Corrosive Substances

Corrosive substances include strong acids like sulphuric acid, nitric acid, hydrochloric acid, phosphoric acid and alkalies like sodium hydroxide, potassium hydroxide *etc.* These substances cause burn on the skin, hence, following precautions should be taken:

1. Bottle should be opened in a fume cupboard.

2. Bottles with bulky chemicals should be handled carefully by holding firmly in both the hands. Do not carry bottles by holding their neck.

3. When using the acids, particularly, place the receiving vessel in the sink.

4. Bottles containing inorganic acids should be kept at one place and away from other chemicals.

5. Acids and alkalies be kept separately away from each other.

6. Acid and alkali spillage on working tables, floor and clothes should be thoroughly washed with water after suitably neutralizing with either weak alkali in case of acid and weak acid in case of alkali.

7. Water should not be added to inorganic acid. Acid should be added to water slowly from the side.

8. It is better to pour the liquid with the help of clean glass rod to avoid spattering.

9. Never pipette strong acids and alkalies with mouth. Always use adopter or rubber bulb or bulb pipette.

10. Bottles containing potassium and sodium hydroxide and their solutions should not be stoppered by glass stopper due to their sticking nature, which is difficult to open without breaking the neck of bottle.

11. Solution of sodium hydroxide should be prepared in cold condition due to the generation of considerable heat.

Handling of Volatile and Organic Substances

For handling of volatile substances like ammonia and organic solvents like alcohol, benzene, chloroform *etc.*, the following precautions should be taken:

1. While opening liquor ammonia bottles, especially during summer season, cool it for some time in a freezer to avoid sudden spurt of ammonia gas accumulated in the bottle.

2. Any compound or reagent containing volatile ammonia should not be opened at a place containing the samples digested with sulphuric acid for nitrogen estimation because sulphuric acid absorbs ammonia.

3. Bottles containing organic solvents should be opened in a fume cupboard.

4. Bottles of organic solvent should be placed in a cool place and away from sunlight.

5. Avoid mouth pipetting of organic solvents. Better use pasture pipette.

6. There should not be any flame in the surrounding area of organic solvent.

7. Though the effect of organic solvents on the body is slow, but maximum exposure should be avoided.

First Aid Treatment in the Laboratory

Chemicals cause injury by:

1. Inhalation
2. Contact with skin or mouth
3. Ingestion
4. Contact with eyes

1. Inhalation

Injury like irritation of throat is treated by warm soothing drink.

2. Contact with Skin or Mouth

Splashing of skin is treated by rapid dilution with water. Further, removal is done with soap and water. Cover with sterile dressing in case of burns. Splashing of mouth is simply treated by washing with water.

3. Ingestion

In case of ingestion of strong acids, dilute with drinking water and then by milk of magnesia. Avoid the use of sodium bicarbonate, which causes distention of stomach by the gas and can rupture the stomach wall.

4. Contact with Eyes

Chemical injury to the eye is treated by diluting with water using gentle stream from the wash bottle.

In addition to the injuries caused by the chemicals, there are chances of mechanical, electrical and thermal injuries, then:

1. In case of mechanical injuries like cuts, wash, dry and cover with sterile dressing.
2. Most haemorrhages can be controlled by firm pressure over the bleeding point.
3. In case of electric shock, best remedy is to switch off the power supply. Avoid using bare hands. Use rubber gloves.

2

Definition of Terms and Explanatory Notes

Normal Solution

A normal solution is one which contains gram equivalent of dissolved substance (solute) in 1 litre (L) of solution and is denoted as 1N.

Normality

The normality of a solution (N) indicates the number of gram equivalents of solute contained in 1L of solution or the number of milligram equivalents of solute contained in 1 ml of solution.

Gram Equivalent

The gram equivalent of a substance is number of grams of the reagent, which in a given reaction corresponds to a gram atom or gram ion of hydrogen.

Gram equivalent of a substance can be different in different reactions, Ex: equivalent weights of oxidizing and reducing agents are different in different medium. Equivalent weight of potassium permanganate ($KMnO_4$) an oxidizing agent is different in acid and alkaline medium.

Equivalent Weight of $KMnO_4$ in Acid Medium

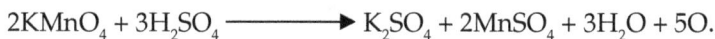

$$2KMnO_4 + 3H_2SO_4 \longrightarrow K_2SO_4 + 2MnSO_4 + 3H_2O + 5O.$$

$$2KMnO_4 = 50 = 10\ H.$$

$$\frac{2 \times \text{Molecular weight of KMnO}_4}{10} = \frac{2 \times 158}{10} = 31.6$$

∴ Equivalent weight of $KMnO_4$ in acid medium = 31.6

Equivalent Weight of KMnO₄ in Alkaline Medium

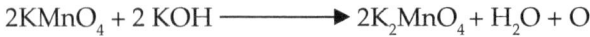

$$2KMnO_4 + 2\,KOH \longrightarrow 2K_2MnO_4 + H_2O + O$$

$$2KMnO_4 \equiv O \equiv 2H$$

$$\frac{2 \times 158}{2} = 158$$

∴ Equivalent weight of $KMnO_4$ in alkaline medium = 158.

Equivalent Weight of Oxalic Acid (Reducing Agent)

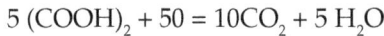

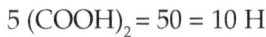

$$5\,(COOH)_2 + 50 = 10CO_2 + 5\,H_2O$$

$$5\,(COOH)_2 = 50 = 10\,H$$

$$\frac{5 \times 126}{10} = 63$$

∴ Equivalent weight of oxalic acid = 63.

Molar Solution

A molar solution is one which contains 1 mole equivalent of dissolved substance in 1L of solution and denoted as 1M.

Molarity

The molarity of a solution indicates the number of moles of solute contained in 1L of solution.

Titre

The titre of a solution is the number of grams of dissolved substance contained in 1ml of solution and denoted as T.

Numericals on Normality, Molarity and Titre

Exercise

(1) 250 ml of a sodium carbonate (Na_2CO_3) solution contains 1.5g sodium carbonate. Calculate the normality and molarity of solution.

250 ml solution contains	= 1.5g Na_2CO_3
∴ 1 ml solution contains	= 1.5/250
∴ 1000 ml solution contains	= 1.5/250 x 1000 6.0 g/Litre
	= 6.0 g/L

Gram molecule Na_2CO_3 = 106 g
Gram equivalent Na_2CO_3 = 106/2
                                     = 53 g

For the Calculation of Normality

53 g Na_2CO_3 dissolved in 1L   = 1N
1 g Na_2CO_3 dissolved in 1L   = 1/53
6 g Na_2CO_3 dissolved in 1L   = 1/53 x 6
Normality   = 0.113N

For the Calculation of Molarity

106 g Na_2CO_3 dissolved in 1L = 1M
1 g Na_2CO_3 dissolved in 1L   = 1/106
6 g Na_2CO_3 dissolved in 1L   = 1/106 x 6 = 0.0565
Molarity   = 0.0565 M

(2) Normality of Na_2CO_3 is 0.025 N. Calculate the grams of Na_2CO_3 dissolved/500 ml.

For 1N   = 53 g/1000ml
For 1N for 500 ml   = 53/2   = 26.5g
For 0.025 N   = 26.5 x 0.025   = 0.6625 g
Gram of sodium carbonate   = 0.6625/500 ml.

(3) Calculate the titre of Na_2CO_3 solution containing 53g/litre.
$T\ Na_2\text{-}CO_3$ = 0.053 g/ml.

(4) Calculate the titre of NaCl solution containing 58.045g/1000ml.
T NaCl = 0.05845 g/ml.

Titration

Volumetric analysis is based on the measurement of two reacting solutions, one of which contains the substance under test and the second is of exactly known concentration (standard solution). The process of measurement of volume is known as titration.

Standard Solution

A solution of exactly known concentration is known as standard solution.

End Point

The process of gradually adding the reacting solution to the standard solution or the reverse, and finding the point at which reaction is complete, is known as end point or equivalence point.

According to the type or reaction that takes place in the given titration, there are several methods of titrimetric analysis. The methods commonly used are:

1. Acid- base titration (Acidimetry and alkalimetry).
2. Oxidation reduction titration (Oxidimetric and reductimetric).
3. Precipitation titration
4. Complexometric titration

Acid-base Titration

Acid- base titration is used mainly for the quantitative determination of acids and bases. Indicators used are methyl orange, methyl red or phenolphthalein. *e.g.* titration of sodium carbonate and hydrochloric acid.

Oxidation-reduction Titration

This titration is used mainly for the quantitative determination of oxidizing and reducing agents *viz.*,

(i) Titration of potassium permanganate and oxalic acid. Here potassium permanganate itself acts as an indicator.

(ii) Iodometric method- Titration of sodium thiosulphate and iodine using starch as an indicator.

Precipitation Titration

These are based on the reactions which result in the formation of a soluble precipitate *viz.*,

(i) Titration of silver nitrate and sodium chloride (argentimetry) using potassium chromate as an indicator.

(ii) Titration of silver nitrate and potassium or ammonium thiocynate using ferric ammonium sulphate as an indicator.

Complexometric Titration

These titration are based on the formation of stable water soluble complex *e.g.* titration of calcium and magnesium salts with disodium EDTA using erichrome black as an indicator.

3

Indicators

The end point is usually judged by adding an auxillary reagent which gives a clear visual change in the solution being titrated. Sometimes the visual change is produced by the standard solution itself. *e.g.*, potassium permanganate. Such auxiliary reagents are known as indicators.

Indicators are weak organic acids or bases. They possess different colour in dissociated or undissociated form and change their colour depending upon H+ concentration. Their molecular and ionized forms are of different colours. Commonly used indicators are methyl red, methyl orange and phenopthalein.

Self Indicator

Self indicators are those, excess addition of which change the colour indicating the end point. *e.g.* potassium permanganate – oxalic acid titration. Here excess addition of potassium permanganate changes the colour and indicates the end point.

I. Theory of Indicators

Example

(1) **Methyl orange**

It is a weak base and ionizes as follows:

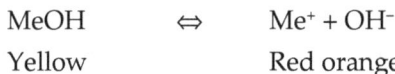

MeOH $\Leftrightarrow$ $Me^+ + OH^-$

Yellow   Red orange

In presence of an alkali due to common ion effect, the dissociation of MeOH will be suppressed and have a colour of undissociated form *i.e.*, yellow colour. However, in presence of an acid, the dissociation of MeOH will

be increased considerably (H^+ and OH form water) and have a colour of dissociated form *i.e.*, red orange.

(2) Phenolphthalein (HPh). It is a weak acid and ionizes as follows:

HPh $\Leftrightarrow$ $H^+ + Ph^-$

(colourless) (Pink)

In presence of an acid due to common ion effect, dissociation of HPh will be less and have the colour of the undissociated form *i.e.*, colourless (Here H+ ions from HPh and from acid combine and the concentration of H^+ will be more, so in order to maintain the equilibrium, the dissociation will be suppressed). In alkaline medium, H^+ from HPh and OH from alkali will combine and form feebly ionized water. Hence, more HPh will be dissociated, with pink colour indicating more concentration of Ph ions in the solution.

Choice of Indicator

For the selection of a suitable indicator, particularly of acid base titration, the chief requirement is the pH range in which indicator changes in colour as close as possible to the pH of unknown solution at the end point.

1. Titration of Strong acid with weak base

Say Na_2CO_3 and HC1

$Na_2CO_3 + 2HC1 \rightarrow 2NaC1 + H_2CO_3$

By this reaction a salt (NaC1) is formed at the end point resulting in acidic reaction at the end point. In such cases, only those indicators are to be used, which change colour at a pH below 7 (Methyl red and Methyl orange). Likewise for strong base and weak acid, Phenolphthalein (HPh) is the suitable indicator. *e.g.* NaOH and CH_3COOH.

2. Titration of Strong Acid and Strong Base (HCl/NaOH)

$NaOH + HC1 \rightarrow NaC1 + H_2O$

Here, NaC1 formed will not be hydrolysed (formed from strong acid and strong base) *i.e.* neutral reaction at the end point. In such cases, methyl red, methyl orange or phenolphthalein can be used.

Details of Indicators

Sl.No.	Name of Indicator	Colour in Acidic Medium	Colour in Alkaline Medium	pH Range at Transition	Preparation of Indicator
1.	Methyl orange	Red orange	Yellow	3.1 – 4.2	0.05g in 100ml water
2.	Methyl red	Red	Yellow	4.2 – 6.2	0.2g in 100 ml alcohol
3.	Phenolphthalein	Colourless	Red violet	6.8 – 8.2	0.1g in 100 ml alcohol

4

Glasswares/Articles in Use and their Cleaning

Beaker (1000 ml) tall

It is made up of glass, spoutless and used for crude fibre estimation.

Desiccator

It is a thick walled glass bowl narrower at the bottom and covered with a ground glass lid. Bottom compartment is filled with a drying agent like fused calcium chloride, calcium oxide or concentrated sulphuric acid. The acid absorbs moisture much more intensively than CaO or $CaCl_2$. Desiccator should be opened only for short period due to hygroscopic nature of drying agent. Desiccator is used for bringing the objects to be weighed at the room temperature without gaining moisture.

Kjeldahl Flask

It is made up of glass, oval in shape at the bottom and having a long neck. It is used for digestion purpose in nitrogen estimation.

Measuring Cylinder

It is graduated and cylindrical in shape, bears a mark indicating its volume and the temperature at which the volume was measured. They are available from 5 to 5000 ml capacity. It is used to measure off a fixed volume of liquid. It should not be kept in oven, because this might change its capacity.

Moisture Cup

It is made up of stainless steel having the shape of cup with a lid. It is used for estimation of dry matter.

Oil Flask

Oil flask is made up of thick glass used for extraction purpose.

Silica Crucible

It is made up of silica, not attacked by reagents, highly resistent to thermal shock because of its very low coefficient of expansion. It is used for ash estimation.

Spatula

It is made up of stainless steel and/or plasitc. It has one end flat and other end spoon like. It is mainly used in handling the sample during weighing. Generally plastic spatula has both the ends flat, used in crude fibre estimation.

Tin Tray

It is made up of Gl Sheet/tin having the appropriate size 6"/9"/½" and used for moisture estimation of fresh green samples of fodders *etc.*

Tong

It is made up of stainless steel having the flat upturned end used for handling the glasswares/articles. Before using, the ends of tong should be cleaned.

Volumetric Flask

It is flat bottom vessel with a long cylindrical neck round which graduation mark extends. The mark indicates its volume and the temperature at which its volume was measured. Flasks are available form 5 to 5000 ml capacities. It is used to prepare solutions. Flasks should not be heated or kept in oven, because this might change its capacity.

Wash Bottle

It consists of a 500 ml thin walled flat bottom flask closed with a glass stopper carrying two glass tubes, one of them is short and is bent at an obtuse angle, which is used to blow air into the flask and it ends directly under the stopper. Other tube is long and extends upto the bottom of flask. The top end of tube is bent at an angle of 60-70° and connected by means of a piece of rubber tube (4-5 cm long) to a short glass tube with a capillary down at its end.

Cleaning of Glasswares

For thorough cleaning, the following solutions can be used:

1. Warm concentrated sodium carbonate solution.
2. Warm alkaline potassium permanganate solution, which is prepared by dissolving 5 g potassium permanganate in 100 ml hot sodium hydroxide solution (10 per cent).

3. Hot soap solution
4. Chromic acid cleaning solution

Preparation

Dissolve 15 g ground commercial potassium dichromate in 100ml hot water. Cool the solution and add 100ml conc. sulphuric acid drop by drop with continuous stirring.

Glasswares are best cleaned with soap solution, because the alkaline permanganate solution attacks the glass. Great care must be taken while working with chromic acid solution because it may cause burns. If some solid particles adhere to the vessel wall which can not be removed by the above cleaning solutions, introduce small pieces of paper into the vessel, add warm water, shake the mixture vigorously and then wash.

Since all the dust and deposition can not be cleaned using the same reagent, there are different reagents/solutions for the same. The deposition of minerals can be removed by using mineral acid (HC1) and their salts by sulphuric acid.

After cleaning with the cleaning solution, wash with tap water 6-7 times and rinse with distilled water 2-3 times.

Drying of Glasswares

After cleaning, the glasswares should be dried prior to their use for analysis. Generally, glasswares are dried in hot air oven at 70-80°C. Pipettes, burettes, volumetric flasks, measuring cylinders are not dried in oven. Burette is dried by keeping the burette on the stand downward. Similarly pipettes are dried by keeping on pipette stand.

5

General Precautions during Weighing

Following precautions are to be taken to keep the balance in working order for accurate results:

1. Sit in front of balance.
2. Keep no object inside the balance case except calcium chloride as moisture absorbent.
3. Don't move the balance after setting. Ensure zero point of the balance before each weighing.
4. While weighing, open only side doors.
5. Never place the substance directly on the pan.
6. Objects being weighed should have the same temperature as that of room. Hence, keep weighing material in a desiccator for 15-20 minutes before weighing.
7. Never load the balance above its maximum limit.
8. Change the load on the balance only after fully arresting the balance.
9. When observing pointer deflections, keep the case door shut.
10. Never touch the weights, pan or balance beam. Handle weights only with plastic tipped forceps.
11. Place the weight centrally on the right and object on the left hand pan.
12. Weights should be placed from larger to smaller.

13. Open the weight box only when weighing.
14. Before and after use, keep the rider on the carrier hook.
15. After weighing, clean the balance with soft brush and put the cover.

6

Preparation of Solutions and their Preservation

Details of Common Acids in Aqueous Form

(Various strengths of common acids, alkalies and other reagents)

Acids	Strength (Per cent by weight)	Specific Gravity (g/cm³)	Normality (N)	Volume ml for IL
Hydrochloric acid	36.0	1.18	12.0	82
Sulphuric acid	96.0	1.84	36.0	28
Nitric acid	70.0	1.42	16.0	63

Determination of Normality of Acids

Formula

$$N= \frac{a \times d \times 1000}{100\, E}$$

a = Percentage of acid

d = Specific gravity

E = Gram equivalent

For Concentrated Sulphuric Acid

$$N = \frac{96 \times 1.84 \times 1000}{49.04 \times 100}$$

N = 36.05 or 36.0

From normality, the volume required for 1 litre is calculated as follows:

N_1V_1	$= N_2V_2$
36 x V_1	= 1 x 1000
V	= 1000/36
V	= 27.77 ml or 28 ml.

Preparation of N/10 H_2SO_4 (Sulphuric Acid)

For preparing 1000 ml of 1N H_2SO_4, take approx. 200ml, distilled water in a 1L vol. flask, and add 2.8 ml conc. H_2SO_4, shake and make up the volume with distilled water. This solution is standardized with standard solution of Na_2CO_3 using methyl red or methyl orange indicator.

Preparation of N/10 HCl (Hydrochloric acid)

Add 8.2 ml of conc. HCl to a 1000 ml vol. flask containing about 200ml. distilled water. Make up the volume upto the mark and shake. Standardize as above.

Preparation of N/10 HNO_3 (Nitric acid)

Take 200-300 ml of distilled water and add 6.3 ml of concentrated HNO_3 in 1L vol. flask. Make up the volume and shake. Standardize as above.

Preparation of N/10 $H_2C_2O_4$ (Oxalic acid)

Weigh accurately 6.3 g oxalic acid. Transfer to 1L volumetric flask. Dissolve oxalic acid in distilled water completely and make the volume upto the mark.

Preparation of N/10 Na_2CO_3 (Sodium carbonate)

Weigh accurately 5.3 g Na_2CO_3 (before weighing, keep in hot air oven for about 30 to 60 minutes). Transfer to 1L vol. flask. Dissolve completely and make up the volume with distilled water.

Preparation of N/10 NaOH (Sodium Hydroxide)

Take a clean dry watch glass and weigh. Weight 4 g of NaOH on watch glass. Transfer the material to 1L vol. flask and dissolve in distilled water. When completely dissolved, make up the volume with distilled water. Standardize against N/10 oxalic acid.

Preparation of NaOH (Sodium Hydroxide) (50 per cent)

Weigh 50 g of NaOH flakes/pellets in a beaker, dissolve gradually by adding distilled water and make up the volume to 100 ml.

Preparation of N/10 KMnO₄ (Potassium permanganate)

Weight 3.16 g KMnO₄ on a butter paper and transfer to a beaker of 1 L capacity. Heat for about 30 minutes. Keep the solution away from light and allow to settle for 3-4 days. Filter through glass wool in to a 1L vol. flask and make up the volume. Transfer to an amber coloured bottle. Standardize against N/10 oxalic acid. The titre of KMnO₄ solution is determined only 7-10 days after its preparation.

Preparation of 5 N HCl (Hydrochloric acid)

Transfer 410 ml of conc. HCl very slowly to a 1L vol. flask containing about 500ml distilled water and make up the volume with distilled water.

Preparation of 1 per cent HCl (Hydrochloric acid)

Pipette out 1 ml of conc. HCl to a 100ml measuring cylinder containing about 70-80 ml distilled water and make up the volume with distilled water.

Preparation of 2 per cent HNO₃ (Nitric acid)

Transfer 2 ml conc. HNO₃ by pipette to a measuring cylinder of 100ml capacity containing about 80 ml glass distilled water and make up the volume with glass distilled water.

Preparation of 3 per cent KNO₃ (Potassium nitrate)

Weigh 3 g KNO₃ on a butter paper, transfer to a beaker of 250 ml capacity. Dissolve by adding glass distilled water. When completely dissolved, transfer to a 100 ml measuring cylinder and make up the volume with distilled water.

Preparation of 1.25 per cent H₂SO₄ (Sulphuric acid)

Pipette out 1.25 ml of conc. H₂SO₄ into a measuring cylinder of 100 ml containing about distilled 80ml water. Make up the volume with distilled water.

Preparation of 1.25 per cent NaOH

Weigh 1.25 g NaOH pellets/flakes on a watch glass. Transfer to a measuring cylinder of 100 ml, add little distilled water to dissolve and make up the volume.

Standardizations of Acid against Alkali or Vice-versa

1. Standardization of Sulphuric Acid/Hydrochloric Acid/Nitric Acid against Sodium Carbonate

Take 10 ml of N/10 Na₂CO₃ in a conical flask of 100 ml, add 2-3 drops of methyl red/methyl orange indicator. Titrate against the acid of unknown normality (acid in burette). Note down the end point and the volume used to neutralize 10ml of N/10 Na₂CO₃. From this volume, the normality of acid is calculated as below:

Acid = Alkali   V1 = 9.8 ml (suppose)

$N_1V_1 = N_2V_2$

$N_1 \times 9.8 = 1/10 \times 10$

N_1 = 1/10 x 10/9.8

N_1 = 1/9.8

From this solution, the acid solution of desired normality can be prepared using the formula:

N_2V_2 = N_3V_3 (desired acid soln)

$\dfrac{1}{9.8} \times V_2$ = 0.1 x 1000

V_2 = 0.1 x 1000 x 9.8

V_2 = 980

Hence, 980 ml of acid solution is diluted to 1000 ml to get 0.1 N.

2. Standardization of Sodium Hydroxide against Oxalic Acid

Take 10 ml of N/10 oxalic in a conical flask, add 2-3 drops of phenolphthalein indicator. Titrate against alkali solution of unknown normality (alkali solution in burette). Note down the end point. From the volume of alkali, normality is calculated by using the formula:

N_1V_1 = N_2V_2

(Oxalic acid) (NaOH) V_2 = 9.8 ml (suppose)

$\dfrac{1}{10} \times 10$ = $N_2 \times 9.8$

$N_2 = \dfrac{1}{9.8}$

Standardization of Potassium Permanganate against Oxalic Acid

Take 10 ml of N/10 oxalic acid in a conical flask, add 10ml of dilute sulphuric acid (1:4), heat upto 60-70°C. Then add N/10 potassium permanganate of unknown normality from burette with constant stirring till there is a change in colour *i.e.* end point. Note the end point. If oxalic acid solution is cooled down, heat it again. (Titration should proceed in hot conditions).

Preservation of Prepared Solutions

Solutions vary in stability due to the contamination with CO_2, exposure to light and heat, growth of moulds, poor quality chemicals and dust. In order to prevent the solutions from deterioration, the following precautions should be taken.

1. Analytical grade chemicals should be used for preparation of solution.
2. Double glass distilled water should be used as far as possible.

3. Chemicals once removed from the original container should never be returned back but stored in another container if necessary.

4. Keep the solutions in properly cleaned containers.

5. Store stock solutions in cool and dark place free from dust and humidity. Unstable substances such as buffers, amino acids, toxins, enzymes must be stored in refrigerators.

6. To take out the solid chemicals from bottles, horn spatula or non-reactive metallic spoon should be used.

7. Photo-sensitive solutions such as potassium permanganate, silver nitrate should be kept in amber coloured bottles

8. Solution of sodium hydroxide should be stored in paraffin coated (internally) bottle as it reacts with glass.

All the solutions cannot be preserved for the same duration and for a long period. So when labelling a solution, date of preparing the solution should always be mentioned.

In order to prepare a standard solution of required concentration from a chemically pure substance, an accurately weighed portion of the substance is dissolved in small quantity of water and the resulting solution is diluted to a fixed volume.

Most standard solutions have to be prepared from substances containing impurities. For example, sodium hydroxide rapidly absorbs CO_2 from the air, being partly converted into sodium carbonate. The concentration of a solution prepared from a weighed portion of such a substance will only be approximate. The exact concentration of such a solution is not determined from the mass of weighed portion, but found by titrating the solution with another solution of known concentration. The process is known as standardization.

7

Proximate Principles in Feed: General View

Main Features of Weende's System of Analysis

For describing various feeds and fodders, Henneberg and Stohmann (1860) at Weende Experiment Station in Germany proposed a scheme of chemical analysis. Under this scheme various nutrients that had some common properties were grouped together and analysed. These nutrients are known as proximate principles of feed and the analysis as proximate analysis. In this system of anlaysis, feed stuff is analysed into 6 fractions. *i.e.*,

1. Water
2. Crude protein
3. Ether extract/crude fat
4. Crude fibre
5. Nitrogen free extract
6. Ash

All the proximate principles are determined by different methods except nitrogen free extract which is determined by difference.

Due to variable amount of water in different samples, results of proximate principles (except water) are expressed on DM basis.

Sl.No.	Fraction	Components
1.	Moisture	Water (Volatile acids and bases if present)
2.	Crude protein	Proteins, aminoacids, amines, nitrates, amides.
3.	Ether extract	Fats, oils, waxes, pigments, sterols
4.	Crude fibre	Cellulose, hemicellulose, lignin
5.	Nitrogen free extract	Sugar, starch, pectins
6.	Ash	Minerals, silica

Moisture

Moisture or water content is most important in a feed. It gives information about the characteristics of feed whether a feed is succulent or dry (bulky feed stuff). Feed stuff containing more than 15 per cent water are not safe to be stored in bulk because there are chances of growth of fungus and mould. Fermentation may also take place resulting in combustion.

Water content in the feed is important, because the relative cost/unit nutritional value is also calculated on dry matter basis. For example: If two types of maize grains are available at Rs. 600 and Rs.620/per quintal containing 15 per cent and 10 per cent moisture, then on dry matter basis, the prices would be Rs. 706 and Rs. 688.80 per quintal, respectively. In this case the maize available at Rs. 620 per quintal and 10 per cent moisture level is cheaper.

Determination of water content is essential, when fodder is to be preserved as silage (for silage making 30-35 per cent dry matter is required). If water percent is less, then it has to be added from outside or vice versa.

The major portion of water obtained by an animal is usually ingested by drinking, but when animals are fed on green fodder containing 75-90 per cent water, the major portion is contributed by the feed. Dry animals during monsoon when on succulent pastures may ingest little or no water. Some amount of water is also available to the animals from the oxidation of feed stuffs *i.e.*, known as metabolic water. One gram of carbohydrate, protein and fat yield approx 0.6, 0.4 and 0.1 ml metabolic water on oxidation. In most of the domestic animals about 5 to 10 per cent water is available through oxidative sources in the animal body. In camel, metabolic water may constitute a major source during summer months. Therefore water content in the feed, determines the water requirement of an animal.

Crude Protein

For estimating crude protein in feed and fodders, nitrogen content is estimated which is multiplied by a factor 6.25 taking into consideration that feed protein contains 16 per cent nitrogen. But the nitrogen content of the proteins of different feeds range from 16-19 per cent, hence different factors are used depending upon the percent of nitrogen in feed. For milk, this factor is 6.38.

Determination of crude protein is important because mostly feed stuffs are classified according to protein content. *e.g.* oil cakes are rich in crude protein.

Similarly, the product from animal sources like fish meal, blood and meat meal are high in crude protein and known as protein supplements.

Leguminous fodders like berseem, lucerne and cowpea are rich in crude protein. By products from cereal crops like wheat straw, paddy straw, jawar kadbi and maize stovers are poor in crude protein content. Protein content of a feed also gives an indirect information about the digestive energy of the feed. Where the crude protein is high, crude fibre is usually low and inturn the digestibility of fodder will be higher.

Proteins are required for various physiological functions *viz.*, maintenance, growth, milk, wool and egg production in the animals.

Ether Extract

The ether extract is that fraction of feed stuff which is obtained when the feed stuff is subjected to continuous extraction with petroleum ether. It consists of glycerides of fatty acid (fats), free fatty acid, cholesterol, volatile oils, chlorophyll, resin and lecithin *etc.* The chlorophyll, volatile oil and resins are not classed as nutrients but found in ether extract of feeds. Since the proportion of components of ether extract will be variable in composition of different feeds, the energy supply from ether extract to the animal will be different. The ether extract in oil cakes would be the fat mostly but in green fodder, large proportion of chlorophyll, volatile oils would also be there. Besides the energy supply, it supplies some of the essential fatty acids like linoleic, linolenic and archidonic acid to the animals which are known as unsaturated fatty acids.

The ether extract content is variable in various feeds and fodders. Green forages are rich in ether extract than by-products of cereal crop residues. Expeller processed oil cake contains 7-8 percent ether extract, whereas, solvent extracted cakes contain very little amount of the nutrient (0.5 to 1.0 per cent). Similarly, solvent extracted rice bran and wheat bran are also poor source of ether extract.

Crude Fibre

Crude fibre includes cellulose, hemicellulose and small fractions of lignin. Lignin is not a nutrient (carbohydrate). The major portion of crude fibre is cellulose, which is highly digestible According to Weende's work, crude fibre fraction represents the undigestible or less digestible fraction of the carbohydrates. At that time rumen microbiology was less understood. It is now known that crude fibre can be as much digestible as the nitrogen free extract. Crompton and Maynard (1938) observed 39, 67 and 28 per cent digestibility in dry roughages, pasture herbage and silages, respectively. Bulkiness of feed is correlated with crude fibre. Bulk for an animal is important, because it gives satisfaction to the animal. Crude-fibre absorbs moisture in the intestine. Since hydrophilic in nature, this character gives the normal distention to the intestinal tract and helps in its peristaltic movement with the result the digesta is propelled downwards.

Crude fibre is the loss on ignition of dried residue remaining after digestion of sample with 1.25 per cent H_2SO_4 and 1.25 per cent NaOH solution under specific conditions. Crude fibre represents a fraction which is composed of (polysaccharides) substances making up the frame work of plants. This portion of food is supposed to be indigested and hence the estimation is based on treating the moisture and fat free sample with dilute acid and alkali, thus imitating the gastric and intestinal action in the process of digestion.

Ash

Ash is the part of feed which remains after ignition. On ignition all the organic matter is oxidised and inorganic matter remains. The part of ash which is soluble in an acid is known as acid soluble ash (inorganic elements) and insoluble portion in acid is known as acid insoluble ash (silica). Higher is the acid insoluble ash in a feed sample, poorer is the quality of feed. Ash component of plant materials is highly variable.

Nitrogen Free Extract

It comprises of starch, sugar, pectin *etc.*

Limitations of Weende's System of Analysis

1. It does not partiton biological materials into well defined chemical constituents.

2. The fibrous fraction lignin is partly dissolved in sodium hydroxide solution and hemicellulose is dissolved by both acid as well as alkali solution. Hence crude fiber may be under estimated and nitrogen free extract may be over-estimated.

Nutritional Significance of Determining the Chemical Composition of Feeding Stuffs

For estimating the nutritive value of feeds and fodders, proximate analysis is the first step. Though the chemical composition does not indicate the availability of nutrients present in the feed stuff to the animals. It gives an information about their quality. Bureau of Indian Standards (BIS) have given specifications of most of the feed ingredients with regard to the proximate analysis. Therefore, proximate analysis would give the information that whether the feed ingredient in question is standard or has been adulterated. Proximate analysis is also being used by the various institutions as well as compounded feed manufacturing plants as a tool for the purchase of feed ingredients in compounding rations.

Basis of Expressing the Chemical Composition

The proximate analysis or the chemical composition of feed stuffs can be expressed in two ways, *i.e.*, on 'as such basis' and 'dry matter basis'. On 'as such basis' means expressing the chemical composition of the feed as is offered and fed to the animals. The advantage of this expression is that it helps in computation of rations. In the later case the chemical composition is expressed on dry matter basis *e.g.* green berseem contains 2 per cent crude protein on as such basis and its dry matter content is 10 per cent, then on dry matter basis the protein content will be 20 per cent. Expressing the chemical composition on dry matter basis has an advantage that various feeding stuffs can be compared among themselves by bringing them at some standard unit of measurement. (Chemical composition is subject of change depending upon various factors).

Other Ways of Expressing the Chemical Composition of Feed Stuffs

According to Weende system of feed analysis, total carbohydrates of the forages are partitioned into crude fibre and nitrogen free extract. This division was based on the assumption that crude fibre is less digestible and nitrogen free extract is more digestible. There is a lot of criticism to this partitioning because neither the crude

SCHEME FOR PROXIMATE ANALYSIS

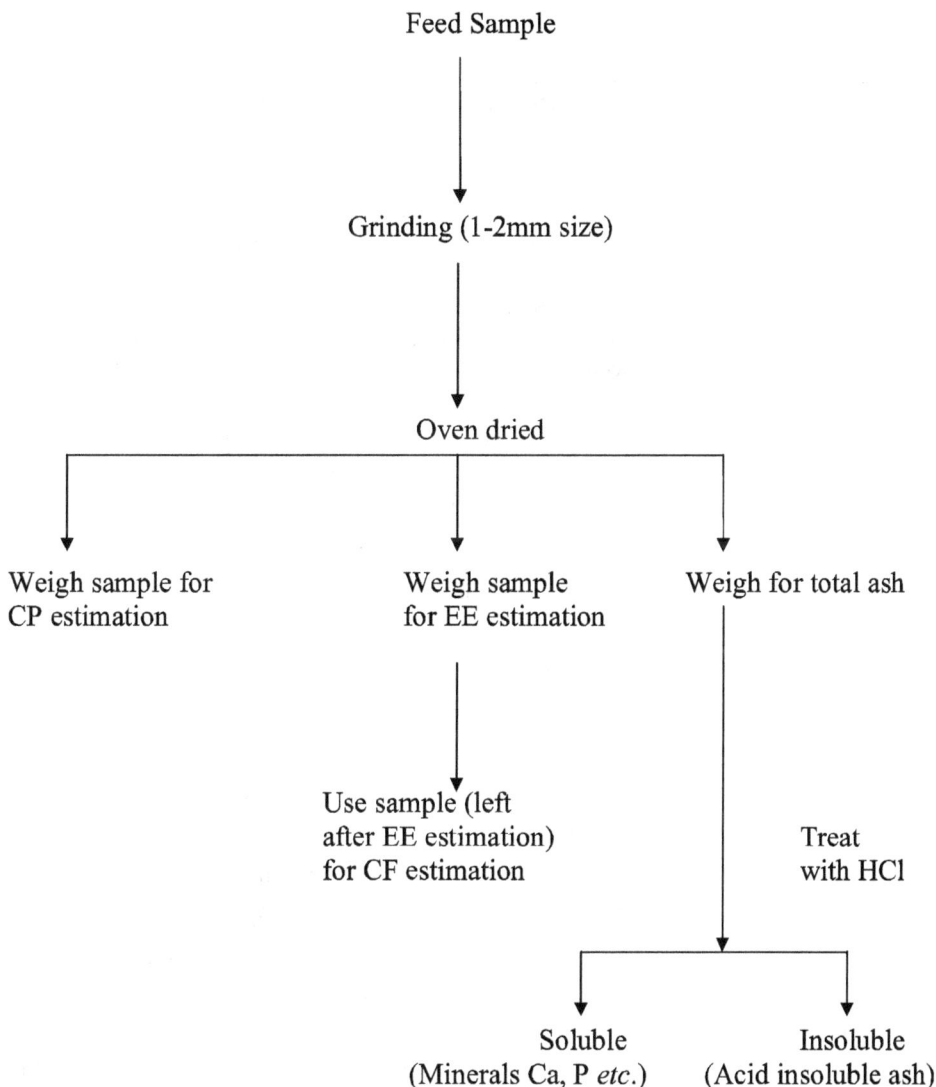

Feed Sample

↓

Grinding (1-2mm size)

↓

Oven dried

Weigh sample for CP estimation	Weigh sample for EE estimation	Weigh for total ash

↓

Use sample (left after EE estimation) for CF estimation

Treat with HCl

Soluble (Minerals Ca, P *etc.*)	Insoluble (Acid insoluble ash)

fibre nor the nitrogen free extract fractions represent any precise chemical constituent of group of constituents. Both vary in composition with different plant species, stages of maturity of plant and conditions under which they are determined. The nitrogen free extract contains lignin also. Knowledge of these limitations associated with the determination of crude fibre stimulated interest in other systems of feed analysis. A number of schemes have been proposed since then. The latest one was proposed by Van Soest (1965) where the whole plant was partitioned into two parts, the one which is soluble in neutral detergent was named as cell contents and the other soluble in acid detergent as cell wall contents.

Estimations by Weende's Method

I

EXPERIMENT	:	**Estimation of dry matter of a given feed sample.**
PRINCIPLE	:	Water content of a feed stuff is recorded as the loss in weight on drying. At 100°C some volatile substances may escape on heating and certain other substances like sugar may decompose. However, the quantity of such decomposable or volatile matters in common feed stuffs is quite small. (Boiling temperature of water is 100°C and heating of a biological material for a certain time removes total water in the form of water vapor Normally it takes 10-14 hours (overnight) in hot air oven at 100°C or in a force draft oven at 60-65°C within 6-8 hours. Representative sample should be spread in tray for 1-3 hours to ensure uniform absorption of moisture from the atmosphere in the laboratory. This is important for the elimination of error due to the absorption of moisture during weighing.
THINGS REQUIRED	:	Moisture cup, chemical balance, hot air oven, spatula, desiccator.
METHOD	:	1. Take a moisture cup, wash it.
		2. Keep in hot air oven for drying (6-8 hours).
		3. Take out the cup and keep in desiccator for 15-20 minutes.
		4. Now, weigh the moisture cup.
		5. Weigh 2 g feed sample in moisture cup.
		6. Keep in hot air oven at 100°C (overnight.) (The lid is kept at the bottom of cup to keep it open for moisture evaporation).
		7. Then remove the cup, and keep in desiccator to bring it to room temperature.

8. Now take the weight of moisture cup containing dried feed sample.

OBSERVATIONS   : 1. Weight of empty moisture cup ——— x g

2. Weight of moisture cup + sample —— y g

9. Weight of moisture cup + sample —— z g

(after oven drying)

CALCULATIONS   : Weight of sample = y-x

Weight of dried sample = z-x

$$\text{Dry matter (per cent)} = \frac{z-x}{y-x}$$

RESULTS   : The given feed sample contains per cent dry matter.

Source: A.O.A.C. (1970). Official Methods of Analysis. 11th ed. Association of official Analytical Chemists, Washington D.C. p. 122.

II

EXPERIMENT	:	**Estimation of moisture in given fresh green sample.**
PRINCIPLE	:	Water or moisture content in fresh green sample is the loss in weight on heating.
THINGS REQUIRED	:	Tin tray, physical balance, hot air oven, scissor.
METHOD	:	1. First of all clean the tin tray and dry in oven.

2. Weigh the tin tray.

3. Now, cut the fresh green sample into small pieces (2-2.5 cm length) with the help of scissor. (While cutting the green sample, no portion should be rejected in order to get material of uniform composition).

4. After cutting, mix the material thoroughly.

5. Weigh 100 g sample in weighed tin tray.

6. Keep in hot air oven at 100°C (overnight).

7. Remove the tray from the oven.

8. Cool and then weigh.

OBSERVATIONS   : 1. Weight of empty tin tray————— x g

2. Weight of tin tray + sample —— y g

3. Weight of tin tray + sample —— z g
(after oven drying)

CALCULATIONS	:	Weight of sample = y-x
		Weight of dried sample = z-x
		Moisture = 100-(z-x)
RESULTS	:	The given fresh green sample contains ———— per cent moisture.
PRECAUTIONS	:	1. Sample should be homogenous.
		2. Sample should be spread in tray in a uniform manner.

Source: A.O.A.C. (1970). Official Methods of Analysis. 11th ed. Association of Official Analytical Chemists, Washington D.C. p. 122.

III

EXPERIMENT	:	**Estimation of crude protein in a given feed sample**
PRINCIPLE	:	Crude protein is actually determined in terms of nitrogen, which is then converted into crude protein. Since average value of nitrogen (in protein) in biological material is 16 per cent on dry matter basis, a factor 6.25 (100/6) is used for the determination of crude protein content. Nitrogen estimation is based on the principle that when nitrogenous compound is digested with concentrated sulfuric acid, ammonium sulphate is formed. Ammonia is liberated by adding alkali to the digested mixture on distillation. Liberated ammonia is absorbed into boric acid and the bound ammonia in boric acid (Ammonium borate complex) is titrated with a standard acid solution. Reactions take place as follows

$$\text{Biological Sample} + H_2SO_4 \rightarrow NH_3 + CO_2 + SO_2 + NO_2$$

$$2NH_3 + H_2SO_4 \rightarrow (NH_4)_2\,SO_4$$

$$(NH_4)_2SO_4 + 2NaOH \rightarrow 2NH_4OH + Na_2SO_4$$

$$NH_4OH + H_3BO_3 \rightarrow NH_4B(OH)_4$$

$$2NH_4\,B(OH)_4 + H_2SO_4 \rightarrow (NH4)_2\,SO4 + 2H_3BO_3 + 2H_2O$$

INSTRUMENTS AND GLASSWARES REQUIRED	:	Kjeldahl flask, chemical balance, spatula, volumetric flask – 250 ml, conical flask – 150 ml, burette – 25 ml, pipette – 10 ml Complete Markham Semi micro nitrogen distillation unit.
REAGENTS REQUIRED	:	1. Concentrated sulphuric acid
		2. **Digestion mixture:** It is prepared by homogenising 20 parts of sodium sulphate and 1 part copper sulphate with the help of pestle and mortor.

3. **Boric acid (2 per cent):** It is prepared by dissolving 2g boric acid in little distilled water and then making the volume to 100 ml with distilled water.

4. **Sodium hydroxide (50 per cent):** Weigh 50 g sodium hydroxide in a beaker, dissolve in little distilled water (keep the beaker in a trough filled with tap water, while dissolving) and then make up the volume to 100 ml with distilled water.

5. **Mixed Indicator:** Mixed indicator is obtained by dissolving 40 mg methylene blue and 100 mg methyl red in little alcohol and then making the volume upto 100 ml with alcohol.

6. **Standard sulphuric acid solution (N/10):** It is obtained by diluting 2.8 ml of concentrated sulphuric acid upto 1000 ml with distilled water in a volumetric flask of 1000 ml capacity. Then it is standardized against N/10 sodium carbonate using methyl red or orange as an indicator.

METHOD : Estimation is completed in 3 stages:1. Digestion 2. Distillation 3. Titration

Digestion:

(a) Weigh accurately 2 g powdered sample.

(b) Transfer the sample to a clean dry kjeldahl flask

(c) Add 2-3 g digestion mixture, 30ml concentrated sulphuric acid and a few glass beads to check the bumping.

(d) Now place the flask in inclined position over a heater for digestion.

(e) Heat gently until frothing ceases, then raise the temperature and digest till the contents are clear (digestion requires about 6-8 hours depending upon the nature of feed sample). At the end of digestion, no black particles remain at the bottom of flask.

(f) After complete digestion, allow the flask to cool.

(g) Prepare the stock solution/extract by dissolving the digested sample into distilled water, transferring into a 250 ml volumetric flask and finally making the volume with distilled water after cooling.

Distillation:

(a) Take 20 ml of 2 per cent boric acid in a 150 ml conical flask and add 1 to 2 drops of mixed indicator.

(b) After setting the distillation assembly, start steaming (add few glass beads to the flask in which steam is formed to check bumping).

(c) Add 10 ml of stock solution to the distillation chamber of distillation unit and then 10ml of 50 per cent sodium hydroxide (Add these solutions after the steam starts coming in the outer jacket of distillation unit.)

(d) Dip the condenser tip into the conical flask containing 2 per cent boric acid and mixed indicator.

(e) Carry out steam distillation vigorously till the ammonia which is evolved, is completely absorbed in boric acid (Distillate).

(f) The absorption of ammonia is indicated by a change in colour from pink to green.

(g) Maintain continuous water supply throughout the process of steam distillation to maintain the temperature of condenser for cooling.

Titration

(a) Titrate ammonia thus absorbed against N/10 sulphuric acid and note the end point.

A blank estimation is also carried out under the same conditions using the same reagents to know the traces of nitrogen, if present in sulphuric acid, used for digestion.

OBSERVATIONS : (a) Weight of sample ——————————x g

(b) Total volume of extract ——————a ml

(c) Volume of aliquot taken ———— b ml

(d) Volume of N./10 acid used for neutralization-c ml

(e) Dry matter of sample ——————-A g

CALCULATIONS :

$$\text{Crude protein (per cent)} = \frac{14}{1000} \times \frac{1}{10} \times c \times \frac{a}{b} \times \frac{100}{x} \times 6.25$$
(as such basis)

$$\text{Crude protein (per cent)} = \frac{14}{1000} \times \frac{1}{10} \times c \times \frac{a}{b} \times \frac{100}{x} \times 6.25 \times \frac{100}{A}$$
(DM Basis)

| RESULTS | : The given feed sample contains——— per cent crude protein (DM basis). |

| PRECAUTIONS | : 1. Liquor ammonia or any ammonia compound should not be kept at the site of digestion, distillation or titration, particularly calcium should not be precipitated in the same room. |
| | 2. Tip of condenser must be dipped in acid to avoid loss of ammonia liberated after the addition of alkali. |

Source: A.O.A.C. (1970). Official Methods of Analysis. 11th ed. Association of Official Analytical Chemists, Washington D.C. pp. 123-128.

IV

| EXPERIMENT | : **Estimation of ether extract or crude fat in a given feed sample.** |

| PRINCIPLE | : When a feed sample is treated with petroleum ether in soxhlet extraction assembly, it dissolves fats and fatty substances *i.e.* glycerides of fatty acids, free fatty acids, cholestrol, lecithin, chlorophyll, volatile oils *etc.* in the sample. On evaporation of petroleum ether, ether extract or crude fat is obtained. |

| THINGS REQUIRED | : Soxhlet extraction assembly consisting of oil flask, extractor and condenser, thimble, cotton, petroleum ether (40-60°C), chemical balance. |

METHOD	: 1. First of all prepare thimble. For this wrap about 8x8cm piece of paper (Whatman filter paper No.1)
	2. Transfer accurately weighed 2 g. sample to the thimble. Plug with cotton.
	3. Place the thimble in the extractor of soxhlet extraction assembly on a pad of cotton.
	4. Weigh accurately a clean dry oil flask.
	5. Connect the flask to the extractor.
	6. Pour the petroleum ether into extractor (More than 1syphon) and then connect it to condenser.
	7. Now start the extraction. Temperature maintained at 40-60°C.
	8. Continue the extraction for 8 hours (condensation rate of 5-6 drops/second).
	9. Now detach the condenser from the extractor.

10. Remove the thimble from the extractor with the help of tong. (Procure sample in thimble for crude fibre estimation).

11. Detach the oil flask, keep in hot air oven for 30 minutes.

12. Remove the oil flask from oven, keep in desiccator for 15-20 minutes.

13. Take the weight of oil flask.

14. Throughout the extraction process, constant water supply is a must to maintain the temperature in condenser for cooling (After the extraction is complete, petroleum ether in the extractor is transferred to a bottle. This is recovered petroleum ether and can be re-used after distillation).

OBSERVATIONS : 1. Weight of oil flask————————x g

2. Weight of oil flask + ether extract ————— y g

3. Weight of feed sample ————————— z g

4. Dry matter of sample —————————A g

CALCULATIONS :

$$\text{Ether extract (per cent)} = \frac{Y-X}{Z} \times 100$$
(as such basis)

$$\text{Ether extract (per cent)} = \frac{Y-X}{Z} \times 100 \times \frac{100}{A}$$
(DM basis)

RESULTS : The given feed sample contains——— per cent ether extract (DM basis).

PRECAUTIONS : 1. Ether extraction should be done for 8 hrs. Preferably to avoid the error due to the duration of extraction.

2. Thimble and sample should not be touched with hands to avoid contamination by lipid or sweat.

Source: A.O.A.C. (1970). Official Methods of Analysis. 11th ed. Association of Official Analytical Chemists, Washington D.C. p. 128.

V

EXPERIMENT	:	**Estimation of crude fibre in a given feed sample.**
PRINCIPLE	:	Crude fibre is that fraction of total carbohydrates which is not digested after successive boiling with dilute acid and dilute alkali. It consists of cellulose, hemicellulose and lignin. It is supposed to be indigested. Hence the estimation is based on treating the fat free sample with dilute acid and alkali.
THINGS REQUIRED	:	Spoutless beaker 1000 ml; measuring cylinder 250 ml, round bottom flask 1000 ml, filtration flask, suction pump funnel, muslin cloth, spatula, policeman, 1.25 per cent sulphuric acid, 1.25 per cent sodium hydroxide, 1 per cent hydrochloric acid.
METHOD	:	

1. Transfer fat free sample from thimble to 1000ml spoutless beaker.

2. To this, add 200 ml of 1.25 per cent sulphuric acid.

3. Bring to the boiling.

4. Before boiling, put a round bottom flask of 1000 ml capacity filled with water on the beaker (it acts as condenser).

5. Continue the boiling for 30 minutes, maintaining a constant volume and rotating the beaker after few minutes in order to remove the particles from the side walls of tall beaker.

6. Remove the beaker.

7. Filter the contents of beaker through muslin cloth. Wash with boiling water using glass wash bottle till the washings are acid free.

8. Transfer the residue back into the beaker.

9. To this, add 200 ml. of 1.25 per cent sodium hydroxide.

10. Bring the contents to boiling. Continue boiling for 30 minutes.

11. Filter the contents through muslin cloth.

12. Wash the residue with 1 per cent hydrochloric acid and then with boiling water until free from acid.

13. Transfer the residue to silica crucible, keep in hot air oven overnight at 100°C.

14. Remove the crucible from oven, keep in a desiccator for 15-20 minutes and weigh.

15. Now, keep the crucible in a muffle furnace at a temperature of 600°C.

16. Cool in a desiccator and take the weight of crucible.

OBSERVATIONS : 1. Weight of sample ——————————x g

2. Weight of silica crucible ——————————y g
+ residue (after oven drying)

3. Weight of silica crucible + residue ——————————z g (after ashing).

4. Dry matter of sample ——————————A g

CALCULATIONS :

$$\text{Crude fibre (per cent)} = \frac{y - z}{x} \times 100$$
(as such basis)

$$\text{Crude fibre (per cent)} = \frac{y - z}{x} \times 100 \times \frac{100}{A}$$
(DM basis)

RESULTS : The given feed sample contains —————— per cent crude fibre (DM basis).

PRECAUTIONS : 1. Muslin cloth should be free from starch and contain 18-22 threads/cm of length.

2. Frothing during boiling may be controlled by using a drop of amyl alcohol.

Source: A.O.A.C. (1970). Official Methods of Analysis. 11th ed. Association of Official Analytical Chemists, Washington D.C. p. 12.

VI

EXPERIMENT	:	**Estimation of ash in given feed sample.**
PRINCIPLE	:	Ash is the residue which is obtained after the ignition of feed sample. On ignition, organic matter is oxidized and inorganic matter remains.
THINGS REQUIRED	:	Silica crucible, tong, muffle furnace, desiccator, chemical balance.
METHOD	:	1. Take a clean dry silica crucible.

2. Weigh the crucible.

3. Weigh 5 g finely ground sample in the crucible.

4. Burn the sample by keeping the crucible on heater (till black smoke stops coming out)

5. Keep the crucible in a muffle furnace upto 600°C for ½ hour.

6. Remove the crucible (after the furnace is cooled).

7. Weigh the silica crucible with ash.

OBSERVATIONS : 1. Weight of silica crucible ——————— x g

2. Weight of silica crucible + sample ——— y g

3. Weight of silica crucible + ash ————— z g

4. Dry matter of sample ——————— A g

CALCULATIONS : 1. Weight of sample = y-x

2. Weight of ash = z-x

$$\text{Ash per cent (as such basis)} = \frac{z-x}{y-x} \times 100$$

$$\text{Ash per cent (DM basis)} = \frac{z-x}{y-x} \times \frac{100}{A} \times 100$$

RESULTS : The given feed sample contains——— per cent ash (DM basis).

PRECAUTIONS : 1. Ash should be weighed quickly, because it is hygroscopic.

Source: A.O.A.C. (1970). Official Methods of Analysis. 11th ed. Association of Official Analytical Chemists, Washington D.C. p. 123.

VII

EXPERIMENT	:	**Estimation of acid insoluble ash in a given feed sample**
PRINCIPLE	:	The residue left after boiling total ash with 5N HCI is known as acid insoluble ash. It contains largely silica.
THINGS REQUIRED	:	250 ml., volumetric flask, Whatman filter paper No. 42, funnel, hydrochloric acid (5 per cent), hydrochloric acid (5 N), muffle furnace, silica basin.
METHOD	:	1. Take 25 ml 5 N hydrochloric acid in a clean pipette.

2. Drop it in silica basin containing ash slowly.

3. Once the ash is wet, the remaining acid in the pipette is delivered.

4. Cover the basin with a watch glass.

5. Digest the contents in silica basin for 20-30 minutes on a water bath.

6. Filter the contents of basin through a Whatman filter paper No. 42 into a 250 ml volumetric flask.

7. During transfer of the contents, give the washings with 5 per cent hydrochloric acid (5-7 ml) each time.

8. After complete filtration, remove the volumetric flask and make up the volume with glass distilled water. (This is known as mineral extract and used for mineral estimation.)

9. Remove the filter paper with residue carefully without any loss.

10. Fold the filter paper, put in the same basin, dry in a hot air oven and then ash in muffle furnace at 600°C for ½ hour.

11. After the furnace is cooled, remove the basin and weigh.

OBSERVATIONS : 1. Weight of empty silica basin ——————— x g

2. Weight of silica basin + acid ————— y g insoluble ash

3. Weight of sample ———————— z g

4. Dry matter of sample ——————A g

CALCULATIONS : Weight of acid insoluble ash = y-x

$$\text{Acid insoluble ash (per cent)} = \frac{y-x}{z} \times 100$$
(As such basis)

$$\text{Acid insoluble ash (per cent)} = \frac{y-x}{z} \times \frac{100}{A} \times 100$$
(DM basis)

RESULTS : The given feed sample contains——— per cent acid insoluble ash (DM basis).

PRECAUTIONS : 1. Volume in flask should be made up only when contents are cool.

Source: A.O.A.C. (1970). Official Methods of Analysis. 11th ed. Association of Official Analytical Chemists, Washington D.C. p. 123.

VIII

EXPERIMENT	:	**Estimation of nitrogen free extract in a given feed sample.**
PRINCIPLE	:	It comprises of starch, sugar and pectin etc and not estimated as such. It is obtained by difference method.
METHOD	:	It is determined by subtracting the sum of CP, EE, CF and ash (DM basis) from 100
CALCULATIONS	:	100 – (CP per cent + EE per cent + CF per cent + Ash per cent)
RESULTS	:	The given feed sample contains———— per cent nitrogen free extract (DM basis).

Source: A.O.A.C. (1970). Official Methods of Analysis. 11th ed. Association of Official Analytical Chemists, Washington D.C. p. 123.

8

Determination of Energy Value of Foods

Experiment

Determination of gross energy of feed.

Principle

Gross energy (GE) is the amount of heat produced from unit feed, when it is completely burnt to its ultimate oxidation products (CO_2 and H_2O). The calorific value of feed stuffs is determined by the wet oxidation of sample with a soln. of potassium dichromate in sulphuric acid. Then energy value is obtained by dividing the amount of 1.5 N potassium dichromate used to oxidize 1 g sample by a factor dependent on the protein content. The technique is simple, rapid, applicable to large number of samples and gives results in good agreement with those obtained by bomb calorimetery. Therefore, it could be suitably used in place of expensive bomb calorimetry for determining gross energy values of feed stuffs.

Reagents Required

1. **Potassium dichromate (1.5 N):** Dissolve 73.545 g of $K_2Cr_2O_7$ in 700-800 ml distilled water in 1L vol. flask and make up the volume with distilled water.

2. **Sodium thiosulphate (0.15 N):** Dissolve 37.227 g of sodium thiosulphate in 700-800 ml distilled water in 1L vol. flask and make up the volume.

Standardize against potassium dichromate. This is always prepared fresh at the time of use.

3. **Potassium iodide soln.:** Dissolve 20 g potassium iodide and 6.4 g sodium bicarbonate in 70-80 ml distilled water in 100 ml vol. flask and make up the volume with distilled water. This solution is also prepared fresh at the time of use.

4. **Starch indicator:** Mix 0.5 g soluble starch with small amount of water forming paste. Bring to the boiling 100 ml of water, add to starch paste with continuous stirring and then boil for 1-2 min. After cooling, this is ready for use. This is prepared fresh.

Method

   (i) Weigh oven dried 0.125 g feed sample (in duplicate).

  (ii) Transfer the sample to a 250 ml vol. flask.

 (iii) To this, add 20 ml of 1.5N $K_2Cr_2O_7$ and 40ml of conc. H_2SO_4.

 (iv) Keep it for 1.5 hr with intermittent shaking. (for oxidation) in dark place.

  (v) Dilute the oxidized material with distilled water and make up the volume.

 (vi) Take an aliquot of 25 ml (1/10) and add 10ml of potassium iodide solution.

 (vii) Store in a dark place for 25 min.

(viii) Dilute the contents to 50 ml with distilled water.

 (ix) The ntitrate (liberated iodine) against 0.15 N sodium thiosulphate using starch indicator (from olive green to green colour).

  (x) Run blank in duplicate in the similar manner as for sample.

 (xi) Calculate the amount of potassium dichromate used for oxidizing the sample by subtracting the above reading from the blank.

Observations

   (i) Weight of sample = 0.125 g

  (ii) Total vol. of extract = 250 ml

 (iii) Vol. of aliquot = 25 ml

 (iv) Vol. of sodium thiosulphate used = Blank-actual reading suppose x ml.

  (v) Value of protein = y

Calculations

GE (kcal/g sample) = ml of sodium thiosulphate used to oxidize l gm sample

$$\text{Oxidation coefficient} = \frac{\text{Oxidation coefficient}}{23.39\text{-}0.069\ P+0.000226\ P^2}$$
(if fat upto 10 per cent)

$$= 24.02-0.1055\ P+0.000621\ P$$
(if fat more than 10 per cent)

P = Per cent protein in dry sample

$$GE = \frac{X \times 80}{\text{Oxidation coefficient}}$$

Results

The feed sample contains————————gross energy.

Precautions

(i) CP estimation of the sample is required.

(ii) Per cent fat is to be ensured.

(iii) Freshness of the mentioned solution at the time of use is to be paid attention.

(iv) Standardization of 0.15N sodium thiosulphate solution is required.

Standarization of Sodium Thiosulphate against Potassium Dichromate ($K_2Cr_2O_7$) using Potassium Iodide (KI) and Starch as an Indicator

Theory

In acid medium $K_2Cr_2O_7$ reacts with KI liberating iodine according to the following equation.

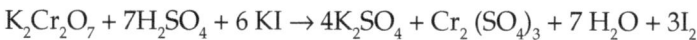

$$K_2Cr_2O_7 + 7H_2SO_4 + 6\ KI \rightarrow 4K_2SO_4 + Cr_2\ (SO_4)_3 + 7\ H_2O + 3I_2$$

The amount of liberated iodine is proportional to the amount of $K_2Cr_2O_7$. Then this liberated iodine is titrated against sodium thiosulphate ($Na_2S_2O_3$) soln using starch as an indicator. At the end point, blue colour formed by the reaction between iodine and starch, disappears and a green colour due to chromic ion is obtained.

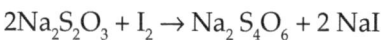

$$2Na_2S_2O_3 + I_2 \rightarrow Na_2\ S_4O_6 + 2\ NaI$$

[The normality of sodium thiosulphate soln. can be determined from the weighed portion used to prepare it, because the water of crystallization of the salt is loosely bound and efflorescence may occur. Hence its composition does not always correspond to the formula $Na_2S_2O_3$: $5H_2O$. A solution of approximate conc. is prepared, which is then standardized against a primary standard.]

Preparation of Standard $K_2Cr_2O_7$ Solution (0.15 N)

Dissolve 7.354 g $K_2Cr_2O_7$ in distilled water in 1L vol. flask and then make up the vol. with distilled water.

Preparation of Sodium Thiosulphate ($Na_2S_2O_3$: $5H_2O$)/hypo solution (0.15 N)

Dissolve 37.227 g $Na_2S_2O_3$: $5H_2O$ in freshly boiled and cooled distilled water in 1L Vol. flask and make up the volume. [On standing slow decomposition occurs causing precipitation of sulphur, especially in presence of sunlight and micro-organisms. Such a soln. is unstable for work]. Keep in dark coloured glass bottle.

Method

1. To a conical flask, add 10 ml dilute H_2SO_4, 1 ml of 100 per cent KI and 25 ml of 0.15 N $K_2Cr_2O_7$ [No iodine should liberate while adding H_2SO_4 to KI. This can be tested by starch indicator].

2. Now add hypo soln. from the burette with constant stirring. A pale yellowish green colour is obtained.

3. Then add 1-2 drops of starch indicator and continue to add hypo soln., till the blue colour of starch – iodine complex is discharged and a light green colour of chromic ions is obtained.

4. Note down the end point.

The normality of hypo solution can be calculated by using the formula:

$N_1V_1 = N_2V_2$

where,

N_1 = Normality of $K_2Cr_2O_7$

V_1 = Vol. of $K_2Cr_2O_7$

N_2 = Normality hypo solution

V_2 = Vol. of hypo soln. used.

Source: O'Shea, J. and Maguire, M.I. (1962). Determination of calorific value of feeding stuffs by chromic acid oxidation. *J. Sc. Fd. Agric.* 13: 530-534.

9

Estimation of Salt Contents in Foods

Salt (Chlorine as Sodium Chloride)

Reagents

1. Silver nitrate (AgNO₃) Solution (0.1N)

Dissolve slightly more than theoretical weight of $AgNO_3$ (eq. wt. 169.87) in halogen free water and dilute to volume. Keep in amber color bottle away from light. Standarize it against 0.1N NaCl containing 5.844 g pure dry NaCl/L.

2. Ammonium thiocyanate (NH₄SCN) Standard solution (0.1N).

Dissolve approx. 7.612 g ammonium thiocyanate in one titre Determine working titre by accurately measuring 40-50ml standard silver nitrate soln., adding 2 ml ferric alum soln. and 5 ml nitric acid (1+1) and titrate with the thiocyanate soln., until the soln. appears pale rose after vigorous shaking.

3. Ferric indicator: Saturated solution of Fe (NH₄) (SO₄)₂: 12H₂O

Method

Weigh 10 g sample and prepare extract with water. (250 ml extract.)

(For this sample taken and to this about 200 ml water added, mixed filtered and then volume made upto 250 ml.)

Take 50 ml extract, add known volume of 0.1N $AgNO_3$ solution more than enough to precipitate all the chloride as silver chloride and then add 20 ml HNO_3. Boil gently on hot plate or sand bath until all solids except silver chloride dissolves (Usually 15 min). Cool, add 50 ml water and 5 ml indicator and titrate with 0.1 N ammonium thiocyanate soln., until it becomes permanent light brown. Substract ml. of ammonium thiocyanate used from ml of 0.1N $AgNO_3$ added and calculate the difference as sodium chloride.

With 10 g sample each ml 0.1 N $AgNO_3$ = 0.058 per cent NaCl

Calculation

Vol. of $AgNO_3$ – Volume of ammonium thiocyanate = x ml

50 ml extract —————— X ml

1 ml extract $\dfrac{X}{50}$

250 ml $\dfrac{X}{50}$ × 250 = X × 5

1 ml $AgNO_3$ = 0.058 of NaCl

X × 5 = 0.058 × X × 5 = per cent NaCl

Standardization of silver nitrate against sodium chloride solution.

Pipette a fixed volume of sodium chloride (0.1 N) – 20 or 25 ml into a conical flask, add 1 to 2 drops of pot. chromate indicator and 20 or 25 ml water. To this gradually add silver nitrate (0.1N) from burette until a persistent red-orange precipitate of silver chromate is obtained.

During the titration, place the flask on a sheet of white paper and agitate constantly. Repeat titration three times, the test results should differ by not more than 0.1ml.

(Preparation of Potassium chromate indicator – Dissolve 10 g potassium chromate in 100 ml water.)

Source: A.O.A.C. (1980) p. 289, 18.034 and 18.035.

10

Colorimetric Method of Estimation of Proteins

Principle

The protein is measured by the intensity of purple colour which results by reaction of -CoNH group of protein molecule with copper sulphate in alkaline medium.

Reagents

1. Biuret reagent: Take 0.75 g $CuSO_4$ and 3.0 g sodium potassium tartarate in 500 ml volumetric flask. Add 250 ml distilled water to dissolve the above solids. Add 150 ml 10 per cent (W/V) NaOH while stirring the contents of the flask vigorously. Make up the volume to 500 ml with distilled water. The reagent can be stored indefinitely. If a black precipitate is observed, the solution should be discarded.

2. Standard Bovine Serum Albumin Solution (BSA): Dissolve 250 mg BSA in distilled water and make up the volume to 25 ml.

Procedure

1. Prepare tubes in duplicate as follows:

Tube No.	BSA Standard Solution (ml)	Distilled Water (ml)	BSA Concentration (mg)
Blank	0.00	1.00	0.00
1	0.1	0.9	1
2	0.2	0.8	2
3	0.3	0.7	3
4	0.4	0.6	4
5	0.5	0.5	5
6	0.6	0.4	6
7	0.7	0.3	7
8	0.8	0.2	8
9	1.0	0.0	10
10	1.0	0.0	10

2. Add 4.0 ml Biuret reagent to each tube and vortex the mixture.

3. Incubate the tubes for 20 minutes at 37°C.

4. Take absorbance at 540 nm against the black. Colour is stable only for 1 hour.

5. Plot the standard curve of BSA.

6. Process the test samples in the same way and determine their protein contents from the standard curve.

11

Colorimetric Method of Estimation of Carbohydrates

Carbohydrates were estimated calorimetrically according to the procedure of Nelson (1944).

Principle

Carbohydrates on treatment with copper reagent and ammonium molybdate reagent give blue colour which is then read calorimetrically at 540 mμ.

Reagent Required

1. **Copper reagent:** Consists of 2 components, copper reagent A, copper reagent B.

   Copper reagent A was prepared by dissolving 25 g Anhydrous sodium carbonate, 25 g Rochelle salt, 20 g Sodium bicarbonate and 200 g anhydrous sodium sulphate in about 800 ml of water and diluting it to a litre.

   Copper reagent "B" consisted of 15 per cent copper sulphate ($CuSO_4$. $5H_2O$) Containing one drop of concentrated sulphuric acid per 100 ml.

   Reagent A and B were mixed in the ratio of 25:1.

2. **Ammonium Molybdate Reagent:** 25g ammonium molybdate was dissolved in 450 ml disttilled water and 20 ml of concentrated sulphuric acid were added to it. 3 g. sodium arsenate (Na_2, $HASO_4$) were dissolved in 25 ml of water. Two solutions were mixed and placed in the incubator for 24 hours.

Procedure

1. 250 mg of the defatted seed powder were digested with 10 ml of 5.4N H_2SO_4 for one hour over a boiling water bath.

2. The contents were neutralized by adding solid sodium bicarbonate.

3. The Centrifuged at 1500 r. p. m. for 10 minutes in a centrifuge. (Nelson, N.J. (1944), *J. Biol. Chem*. 153:375.)

4. The supernatant was transferred into a 100 ml volumetric flask.

5. The residue was washed several times with distilled water, centrifuged and the supernatants were transferred to the original volumetric flask.

6. The residue (negative to Molisch's test) was discarded and the combined supernatant was made upto 100 ml.

7. Take 3 tubes: (1) Test. 1ml diluted digest; (2) Standard. 1ml containing 100 μgm glucose; (3) Blank. 1ml distilled water

8. Add 2 ml copper reagent to the 3 tubes. Heat on a boiling water bath for 15 minutes.

9. Cool, add 2 ml ammonium molybdate reagent and 5 ml distilled water.

10. The contents of all the tubes were shaken, first gently and then by inversion to ensure complete colour development,

11. Read blue colour in colorimeter at 540 mμ.

12

Paper Chromatography and Thin Layer Chromatography

Paper Chromatography

Paper chromatography can be defined as the technique in which analysis of an unknown substance is carried out mainly by the flow of solvent on specially designed filter paper. One of the two solvents is immiscible/partially missible in other solvent. The separation is affected by the differential migration of the mixture of substances. This takes place as a result of differences in partition coefficients.

Principle

When a drop of the sample solution is introduced at some point, migration takes place as a result of flow by a mobile phase (developer). Movement of developer is caused by capillary forces. When the movement of mobile phase is in upward direction, it is known as **Ascending Development** and when it is in downward direction it is known as **Descending Development.**

Ascending development is the simplest of all the methods and is used for quick analysis of large no of substances. It consists in dipping the lower end of paper containing spots in the solvent, so that it is above the solvent depth and then allowing it to rise up the paper by capillary action. The two ends of paper are not allowed to touch with each other. They are kept apart either by clipping. The rate of movement of solvent becomes slower with the increasing height and this slowness in the rate provides enough time for partition equilibrium between two phases to take place.

In descending development, the solvent is kept in a trough at the top which is usually made of inert material. Paper is then placed in the solvent and lid is covered at the top. The rate of flow of mobile phase is more rapid as compared to ascending development. Two dimensional chromatography cannot be carried out by this method (because paper must be cut to fix into the through).

The ratio of the distance, the substance moves compared with the distance reached by the solvent front both measured from the point of application of the sample is termed as RF (Rate of flow).

Types of Papers

Whatman filter paper (α -cellulose 98.99 per cent, β-cellulose – 0.3-1.0 per cent, pentosans - 0.4-0.8 per cent, ether soluble matter – 0.015-0.02 per cent and ash -0.07 to 0.1 per cent) has extensively been used in paper chromatography. The choice of paper depends upon thickness, flow rate and purity. For example – Whatman No. 4 is used when speed of development is taken into consideration, No. 3, when a thick grade for heavier loading is needed and No. 20 is suitable when a good resolution is required.

Proper shape of paper facilitates better resolution. Paper should be washed before use (for removing the reducing substances)

Choice of Solvents

Stationary phases used are classified as follows:

(i) **Aqueous Stationary Phase:** Water equilibrated paper is attained by suspending the paper in a closed chamber, whose atmosphere is saturated with water.

(ii) **Hydrophilic Stationary Phase:** An organic solvent can be used for hydrophilic stationary phase. Methanol, formamide, glycol, glycerol *etc.* are the common hydrophilic solvents.

(iii) **Hydrophobic Stationary Phase:** Solvents like kerosene, aromatic and aliphatic hydrocarbons are used.

Mobile Phase

Mixtures of 2, 3 or more solvent, solutions of salts and solutions of buffer are generally used *e.g.*, Isopropanol- ammonia – water (9:1:2), n-butanol- acetic acid water (4:1:5).

The choice of solvents depends on the nature of the substance to be separated. Minimum no. of solvents and in specified ratios should be used. It makes the chamber saturated with the solvent, which prevents evaporation from the paper during developing.

Preparation of Sample

If the sample is in solid from it should be dissolved in a volatile solvent and the minimum amount of this solution is then applied on the paper by suitable means. Diffusion through the paper is avoided, otherwise it results in large zones.

Technique

The method of paper chromatography may be one dimensional or two dimensional depending upon the type of complexity involved in the analysis.

One-dimensional Chromatography

A strip of filter paper (15-30 cm long, 1 to several cms wide) is laid first. A drop of sample soln. in placed in the centre (1″ from one end of paper) and its position is marked by the pencil. The original solvent is allowed to evaporate in order to make the spot dry. The portion of paper nearest to the sample sport is then brought in contact with a suitable solvent developer. Both paper and developer are sealed in container to prevent loss by evaporation. After some time liquid rises up the strip by capillary action, carrying the constituents of sample along with it at various speeds, according to their partition coefficients. After the liquid had traversed the length of the strip, paper is removed and dried. Time required for the development with butanol acetic acid system is about 18 hrs. The position of the solvent front is marked with a pencil at the two edges of the paper and so called chromatogram is the dried by keeping in an oven or over the hot plate for few minutes. Drying is best carried out by a fan or hair drier (Drying is essential so that the solvents are completely dried from the paper).

The finished dried paper thus obtained is known as paper chromatogram. The position of various constituents on this developed chromatogram is then determined by any physical/chemical method. If the substances are coloured, no difficulty arises, but in case of colourelss substances, several methods have been described for locating the spots.

A number of physical methods have been used to locate the substances and infact physical methods are more advantageous than chemical methods (because the substances on the paper are not converted into other compounds). If the compounds are invisible in ordinary light, ultraviolet lamp can be used to locate the position of the spot.

Chemical methods are used where physical methods cannot be used. Reagents, which form compounds in presence of certain functional groups are available for this purpose. For example:- location of amino acids can be made by ninhydrin solution, which causes the development of blue stain. The chemicals thus used are known as locating reagents. Solids like K_2CrO_4 and liquids like water, methyl ethyl and n-butyl alcohols are mostly used.

The locating reagents are either applied by spraying the soln. of the paper and/ or dipping the paper into the reagent solution.

In spraying method locating reagent is allowed to spray on the paper uniformly by a glass sprayer.

In dipping method, a solvent is first taken in which the substances are insoluble and dipping is then carried on in a trough. Volatile solvents are most suitable for the purpose (they can easily be evaporated off from chromatogram).

Much spraying should be avoided, the result is diffuseness of spots.

Individual components can be characterized by the RF values (rate of flow), where

$$RF = \frac{\text{Distance moved by the component}}{\text{Distance moved by the solvent}}$$

RF value depends on various factors:

(i) The nature of the solvent

(ii) The medium used for the separation or the quality of filter paper used.

(iii) The nature of mixture to be separated.

(iv) The temperature.

(v) The size of container in which the experiment is performed.

RF value can be compared by keeping the above factors as constant as possible.

Applications of Paper Chromatography

Paper chromatography has been used widely for quantitative analysis of inorganic, organic and biochemical interest *e.g.*, for the analysis of mixture of amino acids and sugars.

Separation of Amino Acids by Paper Chromatography (Circular)

Principle

In this chromatography, sample is spotted on the paper, eluted and subsequently visualized by reaction with ninhydrin to form purple colour. Qualitative identification may be carried out by calculating RF value for each spot. Quantitative identification is made by comparing the intensity of colour with standard.

Method

Prepare solutions of 0.1g/100 ml each of known amino acid (4 to 5). New take 8 x 10 inch sheet of Whatman filter paper No. 1 and place equally spaced small circles with a pencil (one for each amino acids) 0.5 inch from the bottom. Label the paper at the top with the name of each amino acid as well as unknown one.

Now roll the paper sheet into cylindrical form (all spots should be on the bottom) and put it into the jar/beaker containing a mixtures of 95 per cent ethyl alcohol and 5 per cent water to a depth of 0.25 inch and cover with a lid/watch glass. Paper should not touch the sides of beaker. Top and bottom of the paper are stapled. Now allow the eluting agent to rises about 6 inch. It takes about 3 hrs. Then remove the paper from the beaker and immediately mark the solvent front position with a pencil. The chromatogram is dried and then sprayed with 0.2 per cent ninhydrin soln. in water saturated with butyl alcohol. Now dry the chromatogram in a oven for few minutes (100-105°C) until coloured spots develop. The different amino acids appear as blue spots. Calculate RF value of amino acid and spots for unknown and finally identify qualitatively the composition of unknown.

Precautions

Do not hold the paper with bare hands, otherwise amino acids will be transferred to the paper, forceps/surgical gloves can be used.

Thin Layer Chromatography (TLC)

The chromatography using thin layers of an adsorbent held on glass plate or other supporting medium is known as thin layer chromatography. Adsorbents commonly used are silica gel, alumina and cellulose *etc.*

Procedure

1. Preparation of Plates

(i) Soak 15 g silica gel in 35 ml water at room temp. The slurry so formed is used for preparing the plate.

(ii) Take clean, dry glass plates (20 x 20cm size) and keep on a plastic board.

(iii) By the help of an applicator, spread the gel material on the plates, thus uniform layer of coating material is obtained (Sometimes finder is added to the absorbent in small quantity before coating *e.g.,* $CaSO_4$ (Gypsum). Thickness of the layer used is 0.25 mm (thicker layers are used more successfully).

(iv) The layers are air dried for about 10 minutes and then activated by heating in an oven at about 110°C for 2 hrs.

2. Method

(i) After the preparation of plate, one drop of sample soln. (0.1 per cent) is applied in a row along one side of the plate, 2 cm from the edge. It is, however, desirable to chromatograph a sample to be analyzed in different amounts, *e.g.,* 1,5,10 µg on one plate. During spotting, layers are covered and protected.

(ii) After spotting, place the plate in a jar containing 0.5-1.0 cm layer of developing solvent (may be chloroform, acetone, benzene *etc.*). A combination of two or more solvents give better result than a single solvent. A typical solvent mixture is *n*-hexane-diethyl ether-acetic acid (90:10:1).

(iii) The chromatograms are developed at room temp (The solvent is allowed to ascent about 10-12 cm above the origin.) Amino acid mix takes 3 hrs. for separation.

(iv) After removing form the tank, dry under warm air for few min.

3. Detection of Spots

(i) The spots are then visualized by the help of ultra violet lamp, or their position is located and detected by the help of some reagents (for colourless spots: - locating reagents are iodine vapour, H_2SO_4 etc.).

(ii) After the spots are visualized, encircle them by pencil and measure the distance the zone and solvent spot travel.

(iii) Calculate RF.

For quantitative work, the spots can be removed, eluted and measure calorimetrically.

Uses of TLC + Applications of TLC

(i) In separating serum proteins.

(ii) In the analysis of urine and blood in pathological laboratories.

(iii) In the fractionation of large no. of compounds.

(iv) In the study of various biological changes *e.g.*, fermentation *etc.*

(v) In the separation of flavaroids of planet.

(vi) Detection of trace pesticides in water.

In nutshell, chromatography constitutes a versatile analytical tool for components like amino acids, peptides, antibiotics, dyes, carbohydrates, vitamins and various fields of inorganic chemistry.

Advantages of TLC

(i) Greater resolving power.

(ii) Greater speed of separation.

(iii) Wide choice of materials as sorbents.

(iv) Easy isolation of substance from chromatogram.

TLC is 50 to 100 times as sensitive as paper chromatography.

Limitations of TLC

It can be used only for small scale preparative work.

TLC is superior to paper and column chromatography.

(i) It requires less amount and is less time consuming.

(ii) Separation is very sharp.

(iii) The capacity of thin layers of an adsorbent in TLC is higher than that of paper chromatography.

(iv) Because thin layers have physical strength, ascending techniques are preferred for this type of chromatography.

(v) In TLC, even corrosive reagents may be coated on glass plates. These reagents will however, destroy paper chromatogram.

(vi) Sensitivity of detection of fractions on the plates in TLC is very great. It is probably due to the fact that individual spots in TLC are much less diffused than in paper chromatography.

13

Use of pH Meter

This instrument is an electrochemical measuring device and so it makes use of electrodes. One pair of electrodes is there - the glass electrode and the reference or calomel electrode. The hydrogen ions generate the potential across wall of one of the electrodes and this potential is sensed and displayed by the electrical device, the potentiometer and the electrical component of the unit is called pH meter. This is the most convenient and reliable method for measuring pH. Actually the electromotive force (e.m.f.) of the concentration cell *i.e.*, the combination of the test solution, the glass electrode (sensitive to hydrogen ions) and the reference electrode, is measured.

The Electrodes

As said above two types of electrodes are used in combination to measure the pH of a given solution and these electrodes differ in their construction and function, and they are given below:

1. Glass Electrode

The lower terminal end of the electrode is a very thin walled bulb measuring 0.1 mm across the wall thickness. The bulb, which is made of soda glass, is blown on a hard glass tube of high resistance. The bulb is filled with 0.1 M HCl per liter and this solution is connected to a platinum wire through silver - silver chloride electrode, which is reversible to hydrogen ions. The silver chloride is present as deposit on metallic silver. When the electrode is immersed in a solution, a potential is developed across the thin wall of the bulb, relative to the hydrogen ion concentration present in the solution. The glass electrode in the sample solution makes only one half of the cell and a reference electrode completes the measuring circuit. Glass electrode is sensitive to hydrogen ions but the reference electrode is not. This part of circuit of cell may be written as:

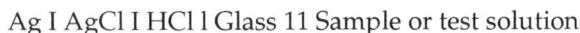

Ag I AgCl I HCl l Glass 11 Sample or test solution

The substances of the left hand side of double line are within the electrode bulb and the double lines represent the wall of the bulb *i.e.* the salt bridge, and on right side of line is indicated the solution into which the electrode is immersed. Thus from left to right it gives the sequence of components from core of electrode to outside. In case of the glass electrode the salt, proteins or oxidizing and reducing agents do not readily affect the potential, and so they can be used with the wide variety of solution-media. The disadvantage is that it is mechanically fragile and the internal resistance of the semi- conductive glass membrane is very high. Since the pH dependent potential is generated across the glass membrane, its thickness should have enough mechanical strength without excessive resistance.

2. Calomel Electrode

These are commonly used as reference electrodes. Electrode is filled with potassium chloride solution, which remains in contact with mercurous chloride and mercury. *Mercurous chloride is known as calomel, and hence the name of the electrode.* This stable electrode is easily prepared and its potential with respect to standard hydrogen electrode is accurately known. The hydrogen electrodes, themselves are highly inconvenient to use, so in practice reference electrodes have substituted them. This part of circuit of the pH measuring cell, in continuation with that of the glass electrode can be written as:

Sample or test solution 11 Glass I KC11 Hg_2Cl_2 I Hg. Here the components are represented from outside to core of electrode, beginning from left hand side.

Many of the models available have the combination electrode that a combination of both glass and reference electrodes but their separate construction is given in the accompanying Figure 13.1.

3. pH Meter

We have learnt that both electrodes along with the solution make a cell and the e.m.f. of this complete cell (E) will be

$$E = E_{ref} - E_{glass}$$

E_{ref}, the potential of calomel electrode, at room temperature *i.e.* about 25° is+0.0250, while E_{glass} depends on the hydrogen ion concentration of the test solution *i.e.* pH_t Then according to Nerst equation, without going in to mathematical details, we have:

$$E_{glass} = 0.342 - 0.059\ pH_t$$

This is because there is a 59 mV change in potential for a ten-fold change in the activity of a monovalent ion as hydrogen. Then,

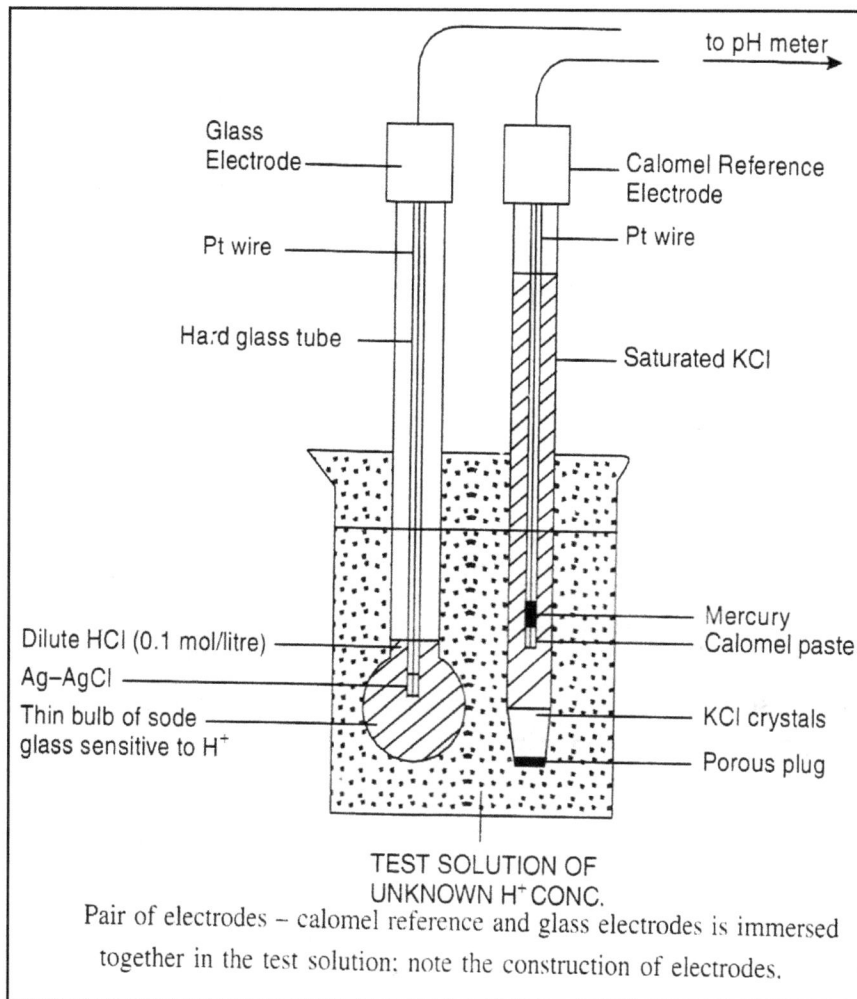

TEST SOLUTION OF UNKNOWN H⁺ CONC.

Pair of electrodes – calomel reference and glass electrodes is immersed together in the test solution: note the construction of electrodes.

Figure 13.1: Pair of Electrodes Calomel Reference and Glass Electrodes is Immersed.

$$E = 0.250 - (0.342 - 0.059 \text{ pH}_t)$$

Or
$$E = -0.092 + 0.058 \text{ pH}_t$$

The above equation is the consequence of the principle that opening of bracket will make - 0.342 and +0.059; then deduction of 0.250, which is a smaller number from -0.342 will yield 0.092.

The glass electrode has a very high resistance in the range of 10^6 to 10^8 O (symbol stands for Ohms, the unit of resistance) and then only a potentiometer of high input impedance can measure the potential.

The Precautions and Care of pH Meter

The pH meters are manufactured in a wide variety of shapes and sizes to suit a particular purpose such for measuring the pH of buccal cavity, blood, flat moist surface' e g. electrofocusing gel), field work testing such as of soil or other ecological components, and even micro-electrodes for intracellular pH. But in all cases the principle of measurement remain the same and so all of them can be operated with little variation as per specifications of the manufacturer.

☆ New glass electrodes must be first soaked in 0.1 M HCl per liter solution or only distilled water for many hours before use. It is important that the outer layer of glass electrode remains hydrated and so they are always kept immersed in a solution. Thin glass membrane is fragile and must be protected from being broken or scratched. It must not be rubbed to clean as that will form the static current. The gelatinous or protein materials must be cleaned from electrode surface because after drying they may cause hindrance.

☆ Preferably the beaker should be on a constant temperature; K_w (dissociation constant for water). pk and pH of standard solution vary with temperature. Though the temperature compensator is prided in the instrument, but that counts only for the variations in e.m.f. of the electrodes with temperature and not for these factors.

The dissociation constant and pH of neutrality at different temperatures.

Temperature (°C)	Value of K	pH of neutrality
0	$10^{-14.94}$	7.97
25	$10^{-14.00}$	7.00
37	$10^{-13.60}$	6.80
40	$10^{-13.53}$	6.77
75	$10^{-12.77}$	6.39
100	$10^{-12.32}$	6.16

☆ Electrodes must be washed with distilled water, before and after being used each time. A thorough w ash must follow the measurement of pH of a solution having biological macromolecules in high concentration.

☆ The pH meter is always calibrated before use with reference to standard solution. The instrument should be calibrated around the expected pH of the solution to be tested and for this pH tablets are provided by the instrument manufactures, which are used as instructed in that literature.

☆ The solution to be tested must be stirred well before pH is measured. For usual classroom practice it can be done with a magnetic stirrer.

☆ Generally the glass electrode is quite sensitive and accurate to low pH values but for strong bases the recorded pH is much due to interference of ions like sodium. Ordinary glass electrode is not suitable for measuring pH beyond 10 and then lithium glass electrode is used. Use of KOH in place of NaOH is recommended for titrating high pH values.

1. For storage, the pH meter is switched to zero reading, but main supply of current is kept on. The electrodes as said above are stored immersed in distilled water so that they do not go dry in any case. If at all they go dry they are to be soaked again and recalibrated for quite a few times otherwise their results remain doubtful.

14
Estimation of β-Carotene

Experiment

Estimation of β-carotene

Principal

The carotenoids in feeds are extracted with the help of a suitable column and then measured in a spectrophotometer.

Things Required

Glass column (30 cm X 1 cm), conical flask, beaker, bell jar, suction pump, spectrophotometer, Whatman filter paper No. 1 and separating funnel *etc.*

Chemicals Requried

Pure beta-carotene, extra pure petroleum ether, acetone (colourless), calcium hydroxide, anhydrous sodium sulphate and alumina.

Method

1. Take 25 g feed/fodder sample in a beaker and mix with 100 ml of acetone – petroleum ether (1:1) mixture.
2. Keep under a bell jar overnight for the extraction of carotenoids.
3. Filter the extract through Whatman filter paper No. 1
4. Wash the residue twice using 50 ml of acetone petroleum ether mixture each time. (More washing may be required for the complete extraction of yellow colour).

5. Take the pooled filtrate in a separating funnel and shake with 50 ml distilled water.

6. Discard the water layer in the bottom.

7. Repeat the washings twice.

8. Dry the solvent layer containing carotenoids over anhydrous sodium sulphate in a beaker and condensed to a final volume of 4 ml under reduced pressure.

9. Separate the pigments in the extract with the help of a alumina column.

10. Prepare an alumina column (10x1 cm) of alumina with 3 per cent anhydrous sodium sulphate.

11. Make the column functional by running petroleum ether through it.

12. Now load the column with 2 ml of conc extract.

13. Elute the beta carotene using a mixture of 3 per cent acetone in petroleum ether.

14. Collect the elute and make upto 5 ml with petroleum ether.

15. Measure its optical density at 450 nm in a spectrophotometer.

16. Draw the standard curve using graded levels of pure beta-carotene in petroleum ether.

Calculations

1 OD is equivalent to 4 µg per ml of beta-carotene in a 1 cm cell path length.

Results

The sample contains ...... beta-carotene (µg/ml)

Source: Pathak, N.N.; Kamra, D.N.; Agarwal, N. and Jakhmola, R.C. (1996). Analytical Techniques in Animal Nutrition Research 1st edn. pp. 52-53.

15

Preparation of Artificial Feeds

Feed represents a large percentage of the cost of production; therefore, diet formulation is a very important aspect of fish production. Diet formulation allows the nutritionist to develop a diet that can be eaten and utilized by the fish to provide an economically feasible level of production. For diets that contain few feed stuffs and in which the nutritional parameters, such as energy and protein, are fixed, the techniques required are quite simple. In such cases use of algebric or Pearson's square method can be utilized. When diets become more complex and the optimum level of production is to be determined, mathematical programming is the technique of choice. For formulation of ration following information is required.

1. Body weight: can be calculated by formula or measured by weighing balance.
2. Nutrient requirement: total nutrient requirement as per NRC.
3. Availability of feed: feed and fodder available in particular area.
4. Nutritive value of feed and fodder.

Objectives

1. To know about the scientific feeding of fish.
2. To acquaint with the actual field situation of feeding.
3. To provide balanced ration to fish in view of production.
4. To make economical use of available feed resources.

1. Formulation of Ration by using Pearson's Square Method

In this method, desired percentage of protein is placed in the center of the square (16 per cent in this example). The percentage of protein in the two feeds is to be put at the left hand corners of the square (8 per cent CP for maize grain and 42 per cent for GN cake). Then subtract (diagonally) the lesser percentage from the higher percentage values and place the answers in the right hand corners of the square (16-8 = 8 is placed at the top right and 42-16 = 26 is placed at the right bottom right).

Example of preparing a concentrate mixture with a DCP of 16 per cent and TDN 70 per cent to have maize grain, G.N. cake, rice bran and wheat bran.

Average DCP of high protein (GNC) =42 per cent

Average DCP of low protein = Rice bran + wheat bran + maize

$$= \frac{6 + 10 + 8}{3} = \frac{24}{3} = 8$$

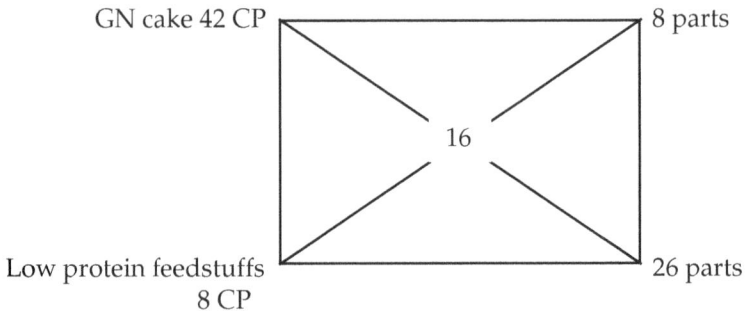

GN cake 42 CP — 8 parts

16

Low protein feedstuffs 8 CP — 26 parts

GN cake and low protein feeds have to be fixed in a proportion of 8:26' for 97 parts (2 parts mineral mixture and 1 part salt to be deducted from a total of 100 parts).

In 34 parts, high protein feed stuffs part are —— 8

In 97 parts high protein feedstuff's parts ———— ?

$$\frac{8}{34} \times 97 = 23 \text{ parts}$$

The amount of low protein concentrate = 97 -23 =74

They are to be mixed in a ratio of 6: 10:8

$$\text{Rice bran} = \frac{6}{24} \times 74 = 19$$

$$\text{Wheat bran} = \frac{10}{24} \times 74 = 31$$

$$\text{Maize bran} = \frac{8}{24} \times 74 = 24$$

Feed Stuff	Parts	Check Per cent DCP Supplied	Per cent TDN Supplied
Ground nut cake	23	x 0.42 = 9.66	0.71 x 23 = 16.3
Rice bran	20	x 0.06= 1.20	0.60x20 = 12.0
Wheat bran	30	x 0.10 = 3.00	0.68x30 =20.4
Maize	24	x 0.08 = 1.92	0.80x24 = 19.2
Mineral mixture	2	—	—
Salt	1	—	—
Total	100	15.78	67.9

Therefore, depending on these calculations, above mentioned parts of feedstuffs can be mixed to formulate a concentrate mixture containing 16 per cent DCP and 70 per cent TDN.

2. When more than Two Ingredients/Feeds are involved

Exercise

A dairyman desires to use a mixture of barley (10.5 per cent CP), oats (12.0 per cent CP) and groundnut cake (42 per cent CP) in formulating a mixture with 18 per cent CP for his animals using barley and oats in the ratio of 2.1. Find out the quantities of each of the ingredient.

Solution

    I. Draw a square on left side of the page.

    II. Put the per cent CP desired in the middle of the square.

    III. Separate the feeds into two groups. Specify the proportion of each feed in each group and calculate the average per cent CP in each group. The weighed average CP in the barley and oat mixture in the ratio of 2.1 would be:

2 barley	:	2 x 10.5 = 21.0
1 oats	:	1 x 12.0 = 12.0
	Total	= 33.0

Weighed average CP (per cent)   = 33/3 = 11.0

    IV. Place "2 barley and 1 oats" with average per cent CP (11.0) on the upper left corner of the square and supplement with its per cent CP (42) on the lower left corner.

    V. Subtract diagonally and record the differences as in the previous example.

    VI. Subdivide the final composite figure for barley and oats by multiplying with 2.3^{rd} and $1/3^{rd}$, respectively.

Barley + oats
11.0   42-18 = 24.0 (Barley + oats)

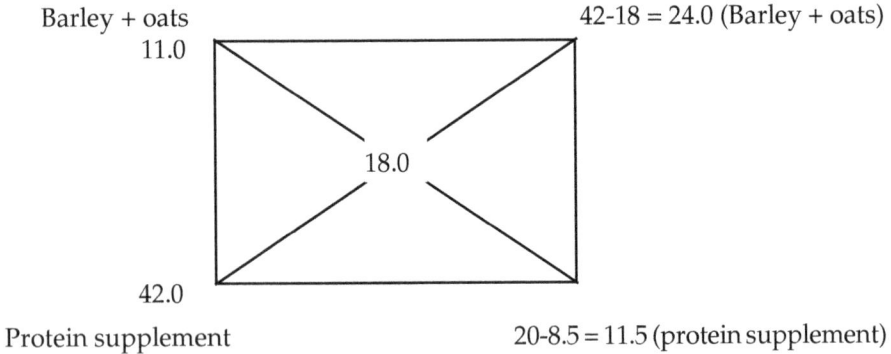

18.0

42.0

Protein supplement   20-8.5 = 11.5 (protein supplement)

$$\text{Amount of barley + oats} = \frac{24}{31} \times 100 = 77.42 \text{ kg}$$

$$\text{Amount of protein supplement} = \frac{7}{31} \times 100 = 22.58 \text{ kg}$$

Total = 100 kg

Out of 77.42 of barley + oats, the amount of barley and oats separately will be Barley = 77.42 x 2/3 = 51.61 kg   Oats = 77.42 x 1/3 = 25.81 kg.

The final mixture will have barley 51.61 kg, oats 25.81 kg and groundnut cake 22.58 kg.

3. When a Definite Percentage of a Particular Ingredient is Involved

Exercise

A farmer desires to formulate a 20 per cent CP mixture for a cow using maize (8.5 per cent CP), oats (12.0 per cent CP) and soybean oil meal (45.8 per cent CP) and a mineral and vita.1min supplement. He wants to include in the mixture exactly 20 per cent oats and 3 per cent mineral, salt and vitamin supplement.

Solution

Under such circumstances, the percentage of maize and soybean oil meal in the remaining 77 parts of the mixture with overall CP of 20 per cent can be calculated as follows:

Since 20 kg of each 100 kg of the mixture is oats so in 100 kg it will supply 2.4 kg CP. The mineral and vitamin supplement will not contribute towards CP. Hence 20 kg oats plus 3 kg mineral, salt and vitamin supplement will supply 2.4 kg protein. So the remainder 17.6 kg (20-2.4) CP should from 77 kg of maize and soybean oil meal. The amount of maize and soybean oil meal in 77 kg can be determined as follows:

Calculate per cent CP needed in the maize and soybean oil meal combination to provide 17.6 kg of CP per 77 kg as follows:

$$\frac{17.6}{77} \times 100 = 22.86 \text{ kg}$$

Then proceed as in the first case

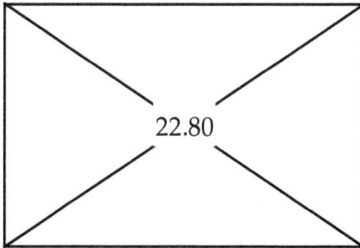

Maize 8.5   45.8-22.86 = 22.94 (Maize)

22.80

SBM 45.8   22.86-8.5 = 14.36 (Soybean oil meal)

Soybean meal = 37.30

On per 77 parts basis

$$\text{Amount of maize} = \frac{22.94}{37.30} \times 100 = 47.36 \text{ kg}$$

$$\text{Amount of soybean oil meal} = \frac{14.36}{37.30} \times 100 = 29.64 \text{ kg}$$

So 100 kg of the final mixture will have maize 47.36 g, soybean oil meal 9.64 kg oats 20 kg and mineral, salt and vitamin supplement 3.0 kg.

16

Determination of Sinking Rate and Stability of Feeds

One of the most important and discussed quality parameters of aqua feeds is their water stability. In the case of fish feed, hydro stability is important because pellets must maintain their physical integrity long enough for the animals to detect and consume them. Poor hydro stability leads to wasted feed and increased organic loading of ponds and effluents, higher feed conversions, and reduced profitability.

Regardless of the method used, hydro stability measurements must provide a quantitative and replicable procedure that eliminates the subjective assessment of quality. Measurable attributes can be used as quality controls to assure that manufactured feeds perform as expected at farms.

Determination of Water Stability

It is carried out by two simple methods

1. Qualitative evaluation
2. Quantitative evaluation

Procedure for Qualitative Evaluation

Take 10 g of pellets in 1000 ml beaker

⇩

Add 850 ml of water

⇓

Gradually stir with magnetic stirrer or hand stirring
for every 10 min for a fixed time

⇓

Look for visual observation (time taken for the feed to disintegrate in water)

⇓

Reporting of the results as water stability in terms of duration (in hrs)

Procedure for Quantitative

Take measured quantity of feed suspended on a 2-3 mm
mesh screen repeatedly immersed or submerged in and out of water

⇓

After particular time, filter the feed through 20 mesh screen

⇓

Dry the residue at 100 degree Celsius for 1 hour

⇓

Compare residual weight to the original wt in terms of percentage

At farms, water stability is often assessed in many different, subjective ways. One is by simply putting some pellets in a glass with water and observing how quickly they disintegrate or how much leaching occurs. Another method is to tie a pellet at the end of a string and submerge it in water until the pellet breaks into pieces or disintegrates. Others use their expertise in chop stick handling to pick up moist pellets to evaluate and determine how pellets maintain their integrity. The reality is that none of the aforementioned methods is a quantitative way to determine water stability. They do not offer a repeatable and quantitative method that can be shared by feed manufacturers and the farmers or biologists in charge of assessing feed quality at farms. The ways to determine water stability used by researchers are more expensive and require special equipment, but yield more accurate quantitative data. The following method is particularly recommended for shrimp aqua feeds.

Sample Collection

Collect approximately 10 g of feed every three or four bags until 20 samples are collected for a particular run. Mix the pellets together by hand to form a composite sample for water stability analysis. Weigh two 25-g subsamples of the pellets and subject them to the laboratory procedure that follows.

Test Procedure

Put 25 g of prescreened pellets with fines removed in an Erlenmeyer flask and add 100 ml of fresh 25° C water. Clamp the flask snuggly in an orbital agitator and run the agitator at 200 rpm for 30 minutes. After agitation, place the pellets on a no. 20 mesh screen and wash the fines off with tap water. This step will remove any fine pieces that disintegrated during the agitation and are smaller than the screen size. After washing, allow excess water to drip off for several minutes. Place the screen in a convection oven for two hours at 130° C, then remove it to cool to ambient temperature. After cooling, record the weight of each pellet sample.

Calculations of Water Stability

$$\text{Water Stability (per cent)} = \frac{\text{Final Dry Weight}}{\text{Initial Dry Weight}} \times 100$$

The percentage number then needs to be corrected for the moisture content of the initial sample. Therefore, it is necessary to know the moisture content of both the initial pellet sample and that of the dried pellet sample. Example: If the initial moisture content of a product is 11 per cent, and the moisture content of the final sample is 2 per cent after drying, adjust both weights to an equal basis. The moisture is 11 minus 2 or 9 per cent.Therefore, add 9 per cent back to the dried product or multiply the final result by 1.09.

- ☆ Sample weight = 25 g
- ☆ Final sample weight = 18.5 g
- ☆ Moisture of initial sample = 11 per cent
- ☆ Moisture of final sample = 2 per cent
- ☆ Water stability = (18.5/25) x 100 = 74 per cent
- ☆ Correction for moisture = 74 per cent x 1.09 = 80.66 per cent.

Sinking Rate

Sinking rate is estimated by observing the time taken by the diet particles to reach the bottom of the water column of 30 cm height. Sinking rate is calculated by the following formula:

$$\text{Sinking rate (cm/sec.)} = \frac{\text{Length of water column (cm)}}{\text{Time taken (sec.)}}$$

17

Effect of Storage on Feed Quality

If storage conditions are not optimum the feeds are damaged. These damaged feeds if induced in compound feeds may cause health and production problems. The factors that are responsible for storage losses can be divided into two groups:

1. **Biotic factors**: Includes insects, rodents, birds and microorganisms.
2. **Abiotic factors:** Includes temperature, moisture, breakdown of produce and type of storage.

Insects

Under Indian conditions the most important insects pests of stored grain are *Sitophilus oryzae* (Rice Weevil), *Rizopertha dominica* (Lesser grain borer), *Trogoderma granarium* (Khappra beetle), *Callosobruchus maculates* (Pulse beetle), *Sitotroga cerealella* (Grain moth), *Tribolium castanium* (Rust red flour beetle), *Oryzaephilus surinamensis* (Saw toothed grain beetle), *Latheticus oryzae* (Long headed flour beetle), *Corcyra cephalonics* (Rice moth), *Cadra cautella* (Almond moth) and *Plodia interpunctella* (Indian meal moth). Out of these 11 species of insects, first five are capable of damaging all kinds of stored material therefore, these are known as primary insects while last seven attack broken/processed/milled food grain so called secondary pests.

After mating, the females begin to lay eggs; under favorable conditions a female lays about 200 eggs in one month. Moths lay their eggs within a few days and then die. Larva emerges from these eggs and it causes the greatest damage to the grain. Larva is converted to pupa and pupa into adult. Pupa is inactive and causes little damage. Pupa stage is 4 to 5 days. This type of development from egg to adult is called metamorphosis and the period is about 1 month under favorable conditions. The multiplication of insects is very fast due to laying large number of eggs and short development time. One pair of insects (male and female) could result in over 1 million individuals within about 5 months. The insect's growth is maximum at 12 to 14 per cent moisture and 21 to 27°C temperature.

Rodents

During storage the rodents not only consume the stored material but also contaminant it with their excreta, hair and dead bodies. Each rat is known to void 10,000 droppings, 4 liters of urine and 5 lacks of hair annually. Each rat eats 8.5 per cent of its body weight/day. The losses caused by rats are estimated to be 2.5 per cent of the total stored products.

Microorganisms

The damage caused by microorganisms in stored products is excessive heat and discoloration. Fungi and bacteria are mostly seed born. Most of the storage fungi belong to *Aspergillus* and *Penicillium* groups and they are capable of producing mycotoxins.

Birds

The losses caused by birds are 0.85 per cent of the stored material. They not only consume food grains, but also contaminate with their excreta and feathers. Each bird can consume on an average 25 g grain/day.

Temperature

A produce can be stored safely even at high moisture content above the safe storage level provided the temperature is maintained low and uniform throughout the storage period *e.g.* cold storage. When temperature rises above 66°C the germination of grains is affected and the biochemical activities in the grain are increased that result into more breakdown of nutrients. Temperature ranging from 20-40°C accelerates the development of insects, but above 42°C and below 15°C the development of insects is retarded. A temperature below 10°C for longer period may cause death of insects. Temperature ranging from 2°C to a maximum of 63°C may influence the growth of storage fungi.

Grains being living matter respire to supply energy for biochemical processes *i.e.*

$$\text{Carbohydrates and fats Respiration} = \frac{CO_2 + H_2O + \text{Heat}}{O_2}$$

In anaerobic conditions complete oxidation of food material does not take place so that incompletely oxidized substances such as alcohol and acetic acid are formed which deteriorate quality of food grains.

When grains are stored, the insect population is rapidly built up in a particular pocket and they respire at the rate of 20,000 to 1, 00,000 times more than that of same weight of grains. Thus, heat is generated which raises the temperature of bulk grain from 38°C to 43°C and moisture content from 11 per cent to 14 per cent. Such heating is known as dry heating and the spot where temperature increased due to development of insect is known as hot spot. This hot spot forces the insects to migrate to cooler area or result in their death. This is known as sterilization heat. At the place of hot spot the moisture content is very high which invites the fungal infestation and increase the temperature from 43°C to 63°C and moisture content from 14 per cent to 18 per cent. This is known as wet heating. The same can be summarized in the given below:

Type of Heating	Moisture Content	Temperature Range	Casual Organisms
Dry heating	11-14 per cent	38-43°C	Insects, mites
Wet heating	14-18 per cent	43-63°C	Fungi

Some facts Regarding Temperature

1. Increasing temperature deep in bulk indicates the presence of insect or mould activity.
2. High temperature in all over storage structure indicates the biochemical deterioration.
3. Combination of high bulk temperature and cold weather indicates that the surface moisture will rapidly increase.

Moisture

In feed and feed ingredients, moisture is present in two main forms *i.e.* water of composition and water absorbed. The quantity of free water (water absorbed) held by the grain product is a critical factor, which plays a vital role in the safe storage of stored products. Free water may be defined as the loss in weight brought about by heating for 24 h at 102±3°C or the amount of water that can be removed without changing the chemical structure of the grain. The amount of water in dry feeds varies from about 5 to 30 percent. Cool and dried grain respired at normal rate, but grains containing moisture above critical level respire fast, liberate more heat which can further increase respiration rate and moisture content. The metabolic activity of grain increases slowly from 11 to 14 percent but from 15-20 percent moisture content it increases rapidly. It is recommended that grain having moisture content above a level in equilibrium with 70 percent RH should not be stored.

Critical Moisture Content for Safe Storage of Cereals at 70 per cent RH and 27°C Temperature

Stored Cereals	Moisture (per cent)
Wheat, Sorghum Barley and Corn	13.5
Oat	13.1
Soybean	12.2
Paddy	15.0

Moisture Migration

In storage the moisture of the grain tend to move from the place having higher vapour pressure to lower vapour pressure to equalize the moisture content throughout the storage. This is known as moisture migration.

When environmental temperature falls below grain temperature, damage may take place at the top center, when ambient temperature rises above grain temperature, damage may take place at the bottom of storage structure.

When the environmental temperature is low, the air coming in contact with wall of the storage structure becomes cold and moves down and the air in grains being hot moves upwards. It carries moisture with it, which is absorbed by the grain at top center and hence the grains there are deteriorated. Reverse is the condition in hot environmental conditions.

Breakdown of Produce

Improper storage conditions results in to break down of produce causing nutrient damage and decreases palatability. The loss is not merely in terms of quantity but also in quality of the feed ingredients. The qualitative loss is attributed to chemical changes in protein, carbohydrates, amino acids, fatty acids and vitamins, which affect the nutritive value of the feeds.

Type of Storage

Bagged grains are stored in warehouses, which are also known as conventional godowns. The storage facility for bulk material is a flat or vertical bin also known as silo. The scientific requirement to minimize the storage losses; the storage facility should be:

1. Moisture proof
2. Airtight
3. Insects, birds and rodent proof
4. Fireproof
5. Should have good aeration system to keep the grain dry and cool.

The losses due to rats, insects and moisture are considerably higher if the storage structures are not rodent, moisture and insects proof. If the storage structure is not airtight, then the stored material cannot be fumigated which results in higher storage losses.

Losses during Storage

Storage is the most important post harvest operation. The losses during storage can be divided into two major categories:

1. Quantitative losses
2. Qualitative losses

Quantitative changes are physical changes in weight and volume, which are easy to measure. While, qualitative changes refers to the biochemical changes which take place in the biochemical moieties of stored material.

Quantitative Losses

Weight loss result from evaporation of moisture, from component parts of product being eaten by insects, rodents and birds; and from allowing quantities spill from the container in which the produce is stored. In some instances weight loss may be converted into a slight gain in weight due to reabsorption of moisture from the air. The weight losses in indigenous bulk storage are low than bag storage. The weight losses in the unsealed stacks are higher as compared to sealed stacks. It has been found that the percentage of grains holed by insects is 2 to 3 times the percentage loss in weight. According to an estimate the storage losses of food grain in India amounted to 6.6 per cent of total production.

Assessment of Storage Losses

The reduction in weight registered over the storage period does not always provide an accurate record of the actual weight loss of produce. The tare allowance on bag and the variation in moisture or oil content of the bag fibers are made. The weight of dust, which may consist of powder from the product, insect and rodent frass plus the weight of any insects present, should be deducted from the weight of the product. Moreover, it may account for a 100 percent increase in weight loss; *e.g.* 3000 bags of maize infested with insects after two years in storage showed an apparent weight loss of 7 percent which increased to a 14 percent actual loss when the dust and insects were removed.

Shortage/Accounting for Storage Losses

Punjab and Haryana Govt., estimated the shortage in bag storage as follows: 0.2 percent per month of storage from September to May in case of wheat, 0.2 percent per month of storage in case of gram and barley; 2 percent during the first month, 2.5 percent during first 2 months, 3 percent during the first 3-4 months, 4 percent during the period of storage exceeding 4 months in case of maize, jowar and bajra. Rajasthan Govt., indicated that the maximum limit for writing off shortage in respect of wheat, stored with the state and central warehousing corporation was 1.5, 2.5 and 3 percent for storage of 2, 4 and 12 months.

Methods for Estimation of Storage Losses

Losses Due to Insects

Any of the following formula can be used for calculating the actual percentage loss:

i) The loss of grain in weight per cent = $\dfrac{(TJKI-IK) \times 100}{UK}$

where,

UK = Weight of 100 uninfested grain,

IK = Weight of infested grain,

UKI = Weight of equal number of uninfested grain.

$$\text{ii) Loss (per cent)} = \frac{(W + G + M)\,100\,(W, + G, +M,)}{S}$$

where,

W, G, M = Per cent (by No.) of weevil led, germ eaten and mouldy grain

S = Weight of 100 good grain in g

Wj, G, M, = Weight of W, G, M no. of weevil led, germ eaten and mouldy grain (g)

Losses due to Fungi

The methods for estimating loss from insects are also applicable to fungal damage. However, when mould occurs a considerable proportion of the grain is rejected. The impact of fungal infestation on loss can be estimated by including the separation of mould damage from other types of damage during the analysis.

Losses Caused by Vertebrate Pests and Bird

Losses caused by such as rodents and birds are difficult to assess directly, since they result in the removal of grains from the store. It is difficult to obtain an accurate estimate without accurate weighing of the grain throughout the season. In captivity the *Rattus rattus* (roof rat) has been found to consume 8-12 g/day, the *Mus musculus* (house mouse) 3-5 g/day and the *Bandicota* spp. (benedicoot rat) consume 25-30 g/ day of food grains and feeds. While eating the rats also contaminates an estimated 10 times more food than they eats with urine, feces, hair and saliva.

2) Qualitative Losses/Biochemical Changes

Biochemical changes are concerned with the major modifications which take place in the biochemical moieties of stored feed ingredients.

Carbohydrate Changes

Alpha and beta amylases attack the starches of the grain and grain products during storage, converting them into dextrin and maltose. Amylase activity in wheat increases during the early stages of storage. Water is consumed in the starch hydrolysis reactions and thus, the dry weight of the products of starch hydrolysis is greater than that of the original. Although this hydrolytic action might be expected to result in significant increase in the reducing sugar content of grain, conditions that favor starch decomposition usually favor respiratory activity also so that the sugars are consumed and converted into carbon dioxide and water. Under these conditions that usually occur at moisture levels of 15 percent or more, the grain loses both starch and sugar and the dry weight decreases. At higher moisture levels, however, active carbohydrate fermentation may occur with the production of alcohol or acetic acid and resulting characteristic sour odors.

Soluble carbohydrates of grain germ stored for 8 days at moisture levels from 9 to 25 percent and temperatures from 29 to 50°C produced characteristic increases of reducing sugars at the expenses of non-reducing sugars.

When damp grains were stored in air, extensive mould growth occurred, and the increase in reducing sugars was only about 1/4* as great as the decrease in non-reducing sugars, owing to the utilization of the former by the mould.

The changes in the di-and trisaccharide contents of grains and byproducts during storage under good and poor conditions indicated that under good conditions, concentrations of various sugars remained essentially unchanged, except for a slight decrease in sucrose content. When the wheat was stored at high moisture contents and temperatures, sucrose, glucose and fructose contents decreased, and the maltose content increased.

Changes in Nitrogenous Compounds Total Protein

In grains stored for 8 years under conditions, which might be used, for long-term commercial storage, crude protein remained unchanged.

Enzyme and Free Amino Acids

Proteolytic enzymes in grain and in organisms associated with grain, hydrolyze the proteins into polypeptides and finally into amino acids. These reactions ordinarily proceed very slowly and are not readily measurable until the grain has reached an advanced stage of deterioration.

Lipids

Deteriorative changes in grain fats or oils may be either oxidative, resulting in typical rancid flavours and odour or hydrolytic, resulting in the production of free fatty acids. Grains contain fairly active antioxidants and the fats in unbroken kernels of grain are rather effectively protected against effects of oxygen in the air. For these reasons, the development of oxidative rancidity is rarely a problem in grain storage, although it is often a serious problem in the storage of grain oils and of milled products, particularly whole grain milled products.

Fats in grain are readily broken down by lipases into free fatty acids and glycerol during storage, particularly when the temperature and moisture content are high and thus favorable to general deterioration. Fat hydrolysis takes place much more rapidly than protein or carbohydrate hydrolysis in stored grain. For this reason, the free fatty acid content of grain has been proposed as a sensitive index of incipient grain deterioration.

Nutritive Change

Mineral Changes

Although mineral matter is seldom gained or lost in storage the availability of phosphorus nutritionally important to animals and man, appears to increase in storage. Most phosphorus in grain is present in the form of phytin, a potassium magnesium salt of inositol phosphoric acid. During the storage of flour and more slowly in the storage of whole grain, phytin is acted upon by the enzyme phytase with the liberation of water-soluble readily available phosphorus compounds.

Carbohydrate Changes

Freshly harvested rice is not digested as readily as rice that has been stored for a time. Fresh rice is said to contain an active alpha amylase that causes the rice to become sticky when cooked. This amylase presumably becomes partially inactivated during storage.

Protein Changes

Although the total protein content of grain as calculated from its nitrogen content is generally assumed to remain unchanged during storage, a progressive though small increase was reported in the protein content of wheat during extended storage. This increase in protein on a percentage basis was the result of a loss in carbohydrates by respiration.

The proteins of wheat, corn and soybeans and their ground products were shown to decrease in solubility and in digestibility by pepsin and trypsin in vitro.

Simultaneously, there occurred an increase in amino nitrogen and a decrease in true protein nitrogen. Wheat containing approximately 11 percent of moisture showed a decrease in protein digestibility of 8 percent when stored in sealed jars at 24°C for 2 years. Corn containing about 12 percent moisture similarly stored showed a decrease of 3.6 percent in protein digestibility in the same time. These changes, as well as changes in protein solubility occur much more rapidly in the milled products of grain than in whole grain.

Good feeding grain is characterized by high digestibility and biological value of the protein by the absence of toxic substances (mycotoxins, fungicides *etc.*) by the presence of lipids which have not been excessively hydrolyzed and/or oxidized and by relatively minor changes in water soluble and fat soluble (specially tocopherol) vitamins.

Vitamin Changes

Cereal grains are generally good sources of thiamine, niacin, pyridoxine, inositol, biotin and vitamin E. they also contain significant quantities of pantothenic acid. Vitamin A activity occurs in yellow com but is practically absent in all other cereal grains.

Wheat containing about 17 percent moisture lost approximately 30 percent of its thiamine in a 5-month storage period. This wheat deteriorated considerably during this period because of its high moisture content. At normal moisture level of about 12 percent the thiamine loss in 5-month period was in the neighborhood of 12 percent.

Studies on rice have also indicated that thiamine is quite stable during storage. Hulled rice stored in straw bags for 4 years retained most of its original thiamine content during the first 2 years but a significant drop occurred during the 3rd and 4th year of storage.

Very little information appears to be available concerning losses of the B vitamins, other than thiamine, found in grain (riboflavin, niacin, pyridoxine, pantothenic acid, para-amino benzoic acid and inositol). But it is generally believed that these vitamins with the possible exception of pantothenic acid are rather stable and are not readily destroyed in unbroken grain under normal conditions of storage. Riboflavin and pyridoxine are rather sensitive to light and may therefore, be unstable in milled products exposed to strong light.

Considerable losses of vitamin A have been shown to occur in yellow com during storage. Com stored in steel bins for 4 years contained less than half the crude carotene of fresh com.

Precautions/Measures for Reduction of Storage Losses

1. The grain/feeds should be properly and reasonably dried before storage.
2. Temperature in the storage structure should be maintained below optimum by aeration to avoid moisture migration and reduce activities of microorganisms.
3. Insects should be kept under control to avoid dry and wet heating.
4. Storage structure should be rodent proof, leak proof and free from dampness.
5. Grain should be reasonably free from foreign matter, which enhances development of insects.

In short, the motto should be to keep the grains/feeds cool, clean and as dry as possible.

18

Estimation of Quality of Fish

I

Experiment

Estimation of Peroxide value (PV) in given fish lipids.

Principal

Rancidity brought out by the action of air is known as oxidative rancidity and that brought about by the microoganism is known as ketonic rancidity in oil. In oxidative rancidity oxygen reacts with fat to form peroxides. The PV value should not be above 10 – 20 meq/kg of fish fat, provided PV has not been lower through extended storage or high temperature exposure.The hydroperoxides have the oxidation potential to oxidize iodide to iodine, which is determined by titration against thiosulphate using starch as indicator. The PV is expressed as milli equivalents peroxide per kg of fat extracted from the fish.

Things Required

Glacial acetic acid and chloroform.

10 per cent Potassium iodide solution: Dissolve 10 g of potassium iodide in 100 ml of distilled water.

Starch solution: Dissolve 1.0 g of soluble starch in 100 ml of water, boil well before use. Prepare fresh daily.

0.02 N Sodium thiosulfate: Dilute from 0.1 N sodium thiosulfate solution on the day of use.

Method

1. Weigh 10 g fish homogenate and add 15 g of anhydrous sodium sulfate to remove the moisture.
2. Extract the fat with 50 ml of chloroform and filter the chloroform extract.
3. Take 15 ml of the chloroform filtrate, add 15 ml of glacial acetic acid and 10 ml of 10 per cent KI solution.
4. Keep in the dark place for 10 min with occasional shaking.
5. Then, add 50 ml of distilled water and 1 ml of starch solution.
6. Titrate the liberated iodine against 0.02 N sodium thiosulfate until disappearance of blue colour.
7. Estimate the fat content in 15 ml of chloroform extract by taking it in pre-weighed beaker and evaporating the solvent in the water bath.
8. Dry the sample at 100°C for 1 hour, cool in desiccator and weigh.
9. Calculate the amount of iodine liberated per gram of fat and express as milli equivalent of peroxides/kg fat.

Calculations

$$\text{Peroxide value} = \frac{\text{Titre value} \times \text{Normality of } Na_2S_2O_3 \times 1000}{\text{Wt. of sample (g)}} \times \text{Dilution factor}$$

Results

The given sample contains...................................

II

Experiment

Determination of Total Volatile Bases

Principal

The method is based on a semi micro distillation procedure. Extracts or solutions are made alkaline with sodium hydroxide and bases are steam distilled into standard acid and back titrated with standard alkali.

Things Required

Apparatus

1. Blender
2. Semi micro distillation apparatus
3. Burette, Pipette, Conical flask

Reagents

1. Trichloro acetic acid - 5 per cent
2. Sodium Hydroxide - 2 N
3. Hydrochloric acid - 0.01N
4. Rosolic acid indicator - 1 per cent in 10 per cent ethanol (v/v)
5. Sodium Hydroxide - 0.01N

Method

1. Weigh 100 0.5 gm prepared sample into a homogenizerwith 300 ml of Trichloro acetic acid.
2. Run the homogenizer to obtain a uniform slurry.
3. Filter or centrifuge to obtain a clear extract.
4. Pipette 5 ml of the extract into a semi microdistillation apparatus.
5. Add 5 ml of 2N NaOH. Steam distill. Collectdistillate in 15 ml of 0.01 N standard hydrochloric acid.
6. Add indicator (Rosolic acid).
7. Titrate the liberated acid to a pale pink end point with 0.01N sodium hydroxide. Do a blank determination.

Calculations

$$\text{TVBN (mg/100 g)} = \frac{\text{(N) 14 (300 + W) x V 1}}{500}$$

where,

VI = Volume of standard acid consumed

W = Water content of sample (g/100 g)

Results

The given sample contains.................................

Source: Pearson's Composition and Analysis of Foods 9th edn.,1991, page 510.

III (A)

Experiment

   Determination of Histamine.

Principle

   Bacterial enzyme decarboxylase free histidine in the muscle to histamine. The concentration of histamine is an indicator of bacterial spoilage. Free histamine is extracted from fish with methanol. The extract is chromatographed on silica gel plates. Histamine is visualized with ninhydrin.

Things Required

Apparatus

   1. Chromatographic tank
   2. Silica gel thin layer (TLC) plates or ready coated plates.

Reagents

   1. Histamine standard (0.2 mg/ml) - Dissolve 16.4 mghistamine dihydrochloride in 50 ml methanol.
   2. Solvent system - Methanol: Cone ammonia (95 : 5).
   3. Ninhydrin spray reagent - Dissolve 0.3 gm ninhydrin in 100 ml *n*-butanol and add 3 ml glacial acetic acid.

Method

   1. Homogenise 10 gm fish with 50 ml methanol and transferwith methanol rinsings to a 100 ml volumetric flask.
   2. Immerse stopppered flask in a water bath at 60°C for 15minutes.
   3. Cool, make upto 100 ml with methanol and centrifuge aportion to produce clear extract for TLC.
   4. Spot extract and histamine solution on TLC plate.
   5. A useful spotting regime is 1, 5, 10 µl of extract and 0.5, 2,5, and 10 µl of histamine solution (eqvt. to 0.1, 0.4,1 and 2µg standard.).
   6. Develop plates in the solvent mixture.
   7. Thoroughly dry the plate with a hair dryer (residual ammonia will react with spray reagent) and spray with ninhydrin reagent.
   8. Dry and gently warm plate with a hair dryer to accelerate colour development.
   9. Estimate histamine level in the extract (µg/µl) by comparison of spot size and intensities with those of standards.
   10. Rerun plate with different quantities of sample extract andstandard if necessary.

Calculations

Histamine in fish (mg/100 g) = Histamine inextract (ug/ul x 1000)

Results

The given sample contains.................................

Source: Lieber, E.R and Taylor, S.L 1978, TLC screening methods for histamine in tuna fish. *J. Chromatgr* 153, 143 -52.

III (B)

Experiment

Determination of Histamine - Alternate method

A. 1 Reagents

    (a) Benzene - *n* - butanol mixture -3 + 2 (v/v)

    (b) **Cotton acid succinate** - Dissolve 5 g anhydrous sodium acetate fused just before use, and 40 g succinic anhydride in 300 ml acetic acidin 500 Erlenmeyer flask. Immerse 10 g absorbent cotton, cut into strips in solution, attach drying tube containing drying agent and heat 48 hrs at 100°C.(flask may be immersed to neck in active steam bath). Filter, wash well with water, HCl (1+9), water and finally with alcohol. Dry in vaccum at 100°C.

    (c) **Diazonium reagent** - Dissolve 0.1 g p –nitroaniline recrystallised from hot water and dilute to 100 ml with 0.1 N HCl. Store in refrigerator. Dissolve 4 gm of $NaNO_2$ in water and dilute to 100 ml. Store in refrigerator. Just before use place 10 ml *p* - nitroaniline solution in ice bath for 25 minutes, add 1 ml of $NaNO_2$ solution, mix and let stand in bath 5 minutes before use.

    (d) **Coupling buffer** - Dissolve 7.15 g sodium metaborate and 5.7 gm sod. carbonate in water and dilute to 100 ml. Store in polyethylene bottle.

    (e) **Barbital buffer** - Dissolve 10 g of sodium barbital in 1 litre water and adjust to pH 7.7 with acetic acid (1+ 15) (about 25 - 30 ml), using pH meter. Store in refrigerator to prevent mould growth. Dissolve any ppt by warming before use (50 - 250 ml bottle of the buffer may be kept at room temperature and replenished from main supply when mould growth is apparent).

    (f) **Histamine standard solution** - Dry Histamine dihydrochloride 2 hrs over H_2SO_4. Dissolve 0. 1656 g dried histamine 2 HCl in water and dilute to 100 ml (1 ml = 1 mg histamine). Dilute 10 ml of this stock solution to 100 ml with water (1 ml = 100 ug histamine. Dilute 5 ml of this dilute standard solution and 5 ml of methanol to 100 ml with water (1 ml = 5 ug histamine. Store in cold. Prepare fresh standards weekly.

(g) 4 - methyl - 2 pentanone (methyl isobutyl ketone). To recover used ketone wash once with saturated sodium bicarbonate solution and 3 times with water, distill retaining fraction boiling at 115-118 ° C and check A at 475 nm.

(h) Benzaldehyde - Chlorine free.

(i) Dilute sulphuric acid - 0.01 M accurately standardized.

A. 2 Preparation of CAS Column

Prepare column by firmly lacing small plug of cotton acid succinate (CAS ca 50 mg) in column by cutting off or blowing out bottom of 15 ml centrifuge tube. Wash plug with 15 ml portions of water and two 3 ml portions of alcohol. Let solvents drip through CAS syringing out column by blowing out last portion of each solvent, using 10 ml syringe with needle inserted through rubber stopper. CAS plugs may be used for months by washing shortly after use with water and alcohol as above and protecting from dust with inverted beaker.

A. 3 Determination

Transfer 10 gm prepared sample to semi micro container of high speed blender, add about 50 ml methanol and blend about 2 minutes. Transfer to 100 ml glass stoppered volumetric flask. Rinsing lid and blender jar with methanol and adding rinsings to flask, Heat in water bath to 60°C and let stand 15 minutes at this temperature. Cool to 25°C, dilute to volume with methanol and filter through folded filter paper. Alcohol filterate may be stored in refrigerator for several weeks (Light powdery ppt separating on storage may be ignored).

Dilute 5 ml of filtrate to 100 ml with water (disregard turbidity). Pipette 5 ml aliquot into 16 x 150 mm glass stoppered test tube and add 1 drop benzaldehyde and 0.2 ml 20 per cent (w/v) NaOH (pH after adding alkali should be about 12.4 - 12.5). Shake vigorously about 25 times. Let stand 5 minutes and add 5 ml benzene - n - butanol mixture. Shake vigorously about 25 times and let stand 5 minutes to separate. If emulsion forms centrifuge. Transfer upper layer with fine tipped tube equipped with rubber bulb to previously prepared CAS column, avoiding transfer of any aqueous phase. Re extract aqueous solution with 5 ml of benzene butanol mixture as before, shaking, letting stand 5 minutes and transferring upper layer to column. Rinse lip and sides of column with fine stream of alcohol from wash bottle syringing out CAS. Wash column with two 3 ml portions water and syringe out. Discard solvents and washes.

Elute histamine from CAS into 25 ml glass stoppered Erlenmeyer by washing down sides of tube with 2 ml 0.01M H_2SO_4(volume and concentration of acid are critical) followed by 3 ml water. Syringe out after dripping ceases.

Cool eluate in ice bath, weighting flask with clamp to prevent tipping and let stand 5-10 minutes. Add 0.5 ml of cooled diazonium reagent and let stand 5 minutes in ice bath. Add 0.5 ml coupling buffer (volume is critical, ostwald pipette is convenient) with continuous shaking or swirling to avoid localized alkalinity (pH after addition of coupling buffer 5-6). Let stand 5 minutes in ice bath, saturated solution with about 0.25 gm powdered $Na_2B_4O_7$, 10 H_2O added in one portion. Shake solution immediately and continuously about 30 seconds to ensure rapid and complete saturation (final pH about 8.6). Let stand 15 minutes in ice bath.

Pipette in 5 ml methyl isobutyl ketone and shake vigorously 25 times. Immediately transfer both layers to 16 x 150 mm test tube and let stand 10 minutes at room temperature to separate and warm up. Transfer upper layer with fine tip dropper to second 18 x 150 mm. glass stoppered test tube containing 5 ml barbital buffer. Avoid transferring aqueous and solid phases if present (transfer need not be quantitative). Shake vigorously about 25 times (pH of barbital buffer after washing about 8.3- 8.4). Let stand 10 minutes to separate.

Transfer upper layer with fine tip dropper to 1 cm cell and determine A at 475 nm against methyl isobutyl ketone. Repeat determination on samples yielding A values > 25 ug standard by diluting 1 ml methanol filtrate to 100 ml with water. Alternatively, aqueous solutions may be diluted 1+ 4 or more with water.

Conduct standard and blank determinations as follows. Pipette 5 ml of 5 ug/ml histamine standard solution into 16 x 150 mm glass stoppered test tube.

Pipette 5 ml of 5 per cent methanol into a similar tube for blank. Add 1 drop benzaldehyde and 0.2 ml of 20 per cent NaOH. Shake vigorously 25 times. Let stand 2 minutes and add 5 ml benzene - *n* - butanol mixture. Follow procedure mentioned above beginning "transfer upper layer with fine tip tube equipped with rubber bulb to previously prepared CAS column avoiding transfer of any aqueous phase"

Subtract blank A from A of standard (A) and sample (A) and calculate histamine as under:

$$\text{Histamine, mg} = \frac{A \times 25}{A}$$

Source: A.O.A.C 17th edn., 2000 Official method 957.07 Histamine in sea food chemical) (A Fluorimetric method - A.O.A.C Official method 977. 13 is also available as another alternative).

19

Nutritional Requirement and Management of Supplementary Feeding in Cultured Freshwater Fish and Shellfish

Feed is the most critical input in aquaculture constituting about 60-70 per cent of total recurring cost. The importance of supplementary feeding has been greatly realized with the intensification of aquaculture from extensive to semi-intensive or intensive farming as the natural food produced through pond fertilization is not sufficient enough to sustain the standing crop of cultured species. Therefore, the use of artificial feeds balanced in protein, lipid, carbohydrate, vitamins, mineral with optimum dietary P/E ratio is required to improve the survival, growth, immunity and reproduction of fish.

The basic knowledge on nutrient requirement of fish is the prerequisite to formulate the cost-effective practical diets of fish and shellfish.

Nutritional Requirements

About 40 essential nutrients are required by fish and shellfish in their diets for its better growth, survival and health.

Protein and Amino Acids

Among the different nutrients in fish feed, the protein is considered to be the costliest one and is essentially required for growth, tissue repair, reproduction and health of fish. It is reported that about 40-80 per cent of the feed cost is due to protein alone. As protein represents the most expensive component in fish feed, it is important to determine the optimal requirement level for growth and survival. The most recent approach to reduce the feed cost is to reduce the protein level a much as possible without compromising growth and health of fish. However, insufficient protein level in the diet results in reduction or cessation of fish growth. On the other hand, if too much protein is supplied in the diet, only part of it will be used to make new proteins and the remainder will be converted to energy.

Protein acts both as structural component as well as an energy source, its requirement for fish is 2-3 times higher than that of mammals. The protein requirement varies from 25-55 per cent for different fish species. The gross protein requirement decreases with increase in age and size of fish. Generally 25-30 per cent protein is optimum for practical diets for herbivorous and omnivorous fishes for pond feedings. However, carnivorous fish requires higher 40-50 per cent dietary protein.

Size, water temperature, dissolved oxygen, pH, and feeding rate are also some of the factors that affects protein requirement of fish. The protein requirement of different fish and shellfish is given in Table 19.1.

Table 19.1: Dietary Protein Requirement of some Finfish and Shellfish Species for their Optimum Growth

Species	Protein Source	Protein Requirement (per cent dry weight of food)
Cyprinus carpio (spawn, fry and fingerlings)	Casein	45
C. carpio fingerlings	Fish meal	54
C. carpio juvenile	Casein	31-38
Labeo rohita fry	Casein	45
Labeo rohita fry	Fish meal and groundnut oilcake	40
L. rohita fingerlings	Casein and groundnut oilcake	30
Catla catla fry	Casein gelatin	47
Catla catla fingerlings	Casein gelatin	40
Mrigal fry and fingerlings	Fish meal and groundnut oilcake	40
Puntius gonionotus	Casein gelatin	32
Ctenopharyngodon idella	Leaf protein concentrate	36
C. idella fry	Casein	42
Trichogaster trichopterus	Casein -gelatin	35
Poecilia reticulate	Casein -gelatin	30
Xiphophorus hilleri	Casein -gelatin	40
Poecilia latipinna	Casein- gelatin	40
Pseudotropheus socolofi	Casein – Fish meal	36-40
Haplochromis ahli	Casein – Fish meal	36

Contd...

Table 19.1–*Contd...*

Species	Protein Source	Protein Requirement (per cent dry weight of food)
Pseudoplatystoma coruscans	Practical diets	46
Tor tambroides	Fish meal – casein - gelatin	48.0
Xiphophorus helleri	Fish meal, hydrolysate, krill meal	30.0
Macrobrachium rosenbergii	Fish meal and groundnut oilcake, soybean meal	35
Channa striatus fry	Fish meal and groundnut oilcake	55
Anabas testidineus	Carcass waste and groundnut oilcake	40
Clarius batrachus fingerlings	Casein- gelatin	40
Tilapia aures fingerlings	Fish/soybean meal	36
T. niloticus fry	Casein/albumin	34-56
Oreochromis mossambicus fingerlings	Fish meal	35

The fish does not have true protein requirement but need a well balanced mixture of essential and non-essential amino acids. Gross protein requirement of a fish is the requirement of essential amino acids and some non-specific nitrogen to maintain metabolic activities. With hydrolysis of protein, about 20 different amino acids are released, out of which 10 are essential *viz.* arginine, histidine, isoleucine, leucine, lysine, methionine, phenylalanine, threonine, tryptophan and valine, which are not biosynthesized but required by fish. The amino acid requirement of all the teleost fishes as percentage of protein are almost similar. The essential amino acid requirement of fish and prawn are given in Table 19.2.

Table 19.2: Essential Amino Acid Requirements (Per cent dietary protein) of some Fish and Prawn Species

Amino Acid	Rohu	Catla	Mrigal	Common Carp	Tilapia	Prawn
Arginine	5.75	4.80	5.25	4.3	4.2	3.7
Histidine	2.25	2.45	2.13	2.1	1.7	0.7
Isoleucine	3.00	2.35	2.75	2.5	3.1	0.6
Leucine	4.63	3.70	4.25	3.3	3.4	1.0
Lysine	5.58	6.23	5.88	5.7	5.1	3.2
Methionine	2.88	3.55	3.18	3.1	2.7	1.2
Phenylalanine	4.00	3.70	4.00	6.5	5.5	1.7
Threonine	4.28	4.95	4.13	3.9	3.8	1.6
Tryptophan	1.13	0.95	1.08	0.8	1.0	0.5
Valine	3.75	3.55	3.50	3.6	2.8	2.0

Lipids

Lipids are important nutrients in the diets of finfish as sources of energy, essential fatty acids and phospholipids. Dietary lipids supply energy and provide essential acids needed for structural maintenance of membranes and proper functioning of many physiological processes. Lipids are almost completely digestible by fish and seem to be favoured over carbohydrate as an energy source.

The increase in dietary lipid levels, must, however, be carefully evaluated as it may affect the carcass composition, mainly due to an increase of lipid deposition. The localization and composition of lipid deposits also strongly influence the nutritional value, organoleptic properties, transformation yields and storage time of fish carcass. Lipid being highly digestible has greater sparing action than dietary carbohydrate or protein and playing a definite role in feed utilization. Excess lipid not only suppresses de novo fatty acid synthesis, but also reduces the ability of fish to digest and assimilate it, leading to reduced growth rate. Again, excess lipid in the diet may also result in the production of fatty fish ultimately having deleterious effects on flavour, consistency and storage life of the finished product. Excessive amounts of lipid in diet also possess problem in feed manufacturing.

Although, a wide range of variations, (4-15 per cent) in gross lipid requirement has been estimated for several species, 7-9 per cent dietary lipids are generally considered optimum for practical diets of carps and prawns.

Fish oil is the rich dietary source of PUFA *viz.* eicosapentanoic acid (EPA) and docosa hexaenoic acid (DHA). As in other vertebrates, fish cannot synthesize 18:3 n-3 (linolenic) and 18:3 n-6 (linoleic) polyunsaturated fatty acids (PUFAs) but fish have a requirement of these two essential fatty acids that are to be provided from exogenous sources. Fish fed diets deficient in two of these PUFAs (18:2 n-6 and 18:3 n-3), usually develop deficiency sign such as retarded growth, low feed efficiency, fatty livers, increased water contents in whole body or muscle, high hepatosomatic index (HIS) and substantial accumulation of 20:3n-9 in tissue polar lipids. Freshwater fish, in general, requires either dietary 18:2n-6 (linoleic) or 18:3n-3 (linolenic) acids or both. Marine fish have dietary requirement of eicosapentaenoic acids (EPA, 20:5 n-3) and/or docosahexaenoic acid (DHA, 22:6 n-3). Dietary phospholipids have beneficial effects on growth and survival of fish and prawn larvae. The essential fatty acid requirements of some fish and prawn species are given in Table 19.3.

Table 19.3: Essential Fatty Acid Requirements of some Fish and Prawn Species

Fish/Prawn	Requirement
Common carp	1 per cent 18:2 n-6 and 1 per cent 18: n-3 or 0.5 - 1 per cent HUFA n-3
Grass carp	1 per cent 18:2 n-6 and 0.5 - 1 per cent 18:3 n-3
Catla	Combination of n-3 and n-6
Magur	18:2 n-6 and 18: 3 n-3
Singhi	18:2 n-6 and 18:3 n-3
Tilapia zilli	1 per cent 18:2 n-6 or 20: 4 n-6
T. niloticus	0.5 - 1 per cent 18:2 n-6 or 1 per cent 20: 4 n-6
M. rosenbergii	HUFA n-3

Carbohydrates

A dietary level of 22–30 per cent of carbohydrate has been found to be optimum for the growth of Indian major carps. Carbohydrates not only serve as the least expensive source of dietary energy but also helps in improving the pelleting quality of practical fish diets. Therefore, some form of digestible carbohydrate should be included in fish diets. Feed cost per unit of fish produced can be minimized by optimal use of low-cost energy carriers such as carbohydrate-rich ingredients, ensuring that the use of costly protein is kept as low as possible. Replacing dietary protein by carbohydrate or lipid energy may result in a higher production per unit spent of costly protein sources such as fishmeal, and the effluent nitrogen can be reduced per unit of fish produced.

The carbohydrate utilization of the fish depends up on the feeding habit, structure and function of the digestive system. The capacity of fish to utilize carbohydrate varied by species and in response to variable such as digestibility and starch complexity. Cold water and marine species generally maintain adequate performance with carbohydrate levels in order of 20.0 per cent. Apart from trout, the tolerance of freshwater and warm –water species is generally higher, up to a maximum of 40 per cent.

The optimum dietary requirements of carbohydrates are 25-30 per cent for India major carps and medium carps, 30-40 per cent for common carp, less than 25 per cent for rainbow trout and 6-15 per cent as gelatinized starch for Salmon species. Carbohydrate levels generally do not exceed 40 per cent in carp diets when the raw carbohydrate is being used. But when the carbohydrate is used in gelatinized form, the level of its incorporation may be increased up to 50 per cent in the carp diet. The commercial diet of prawns normally contains 35-40 per cent carbohydrates.

Energy

Energy is defined as the capacity to work, but in biological definition, it refers to muscles activity, energy for chemical reactions in body, to enable movement of molecules against a concentration gradient and for other biological as well as physiological functions in the body. Fish do have a low energy requirement because no energy expenditure is involved for maintenance of body temperature and due to its neutral buoyancy. Other explanations for low energy requirements are less muscle activity to maintain their position as many fishes have swim bladders and less energy expenditure for excretion of ammonia, which is 85 per cent of metabolic wastes that are excreted directly through gills into surrounding water. Physical activities like swimming, escaping from predators and stress, temperature, size, growth rate, species and food are some of the factors that affect energy requirements of fish. Proteins, lipid and carbohydrates contain 5.6, 9.4 and 4.1 kcal of GE/g respectively.

Reference

This portion has been taken from: Training manual (summer school) on Aquaculture diversification towards boosting pond productivity and farm income (08 -28 July, 2015). Organized by ICAR – Central Institute of Freshwater Aquaculture, Bhubaneswar (Odisha), India.

Appendix

Nutritive Value of Feed and Fooders

Ingredient	Average Composition (Per cent)						
	H_2O	CP	EE	CF	Ash	Ca	P
Plant ingredients							
Barley grain	12.8	10.5	1.4	1.9	2.1	0.06	0.33
Corn grain	12.0	7.8	3.8	1.9	1.2	0.04	0.24
Distillers grains (w)	41.8	6.2	2.2	5.6	3.1	0.12	0.12
Oat grain	7.7	10.0	4.2	11.3	5.1	0.07	0.27
Pea, seed	11.8	20.2	1.4	5.5	2.4	0.22	0.26
Rapeseed meal	8.0	30.0	12.0	9.7	8.0	0.67	1.07
Rapeseed oil	–	–	100	–	–	–	–
Sesame oil cake	8.6	25.7	10.2	10.0	6.1	0.49	0.67
Soybean meal	9.3	40.8	5.7	5.3	6.3	0.22	0.56
Soybean oil	–	–	100	–	–	–	–
Sunflower seed meal	7.3	31.6	8.9	24.0	6.4	0.26	1.16
Wheat grain	12.6	10.3	1.4	2.2	2.2	0.07	0.39
Wheat bran	11.6	12.8	3.1	8.6	4.5	0.10	0.89
Wheat flour	12.8	10.6	1.2	0.4	0.8	0.04	0.15
Animal ingredients							
Blood meal	10.8	73.5	0.4	–	5.8	0.14	0.06
Cattle stomach meal	8.3	15.2	2.2	27.2	16.2	1.14	0.18
Fat (pig)	–	–	100	–	–	–	–
Fat (fish oil)	–	–	100	–	–	–	–
Fish meal (peruvian)	9.1	64.2	3.2	–	–	2.38	2.27
Feather meal	9.1	74.5	2.1	0.2	1.9	0.43	0.07
Liver meal	5.6	61.2	20.1	–	3.0	0.14	1.22
Lung meal	5.6	30.0	22.8	–	10.3	1.42	1.17
Meat and bone meal	5.5	38.3	9.8	0.5	25.9	13.3	6.37
Animal feeds							
Poultry feed	11.48	12.30	1.95	–	7.14	0.89	0.21
Pig feed	8.78	12.11	2.52	–	5.06	0.22	0.50
Cattle feed	9.03	15.83	3.82	–	6.69	0.80	0.50
Sheep feed	9.02	10.11	2.28	–	10.18	2.14	0.35
Rabbit feed	9.14	12.16	2.40	–	4.91	0.49	0.69

www.ingramcontent.com/pod-product-compliance
Lightning Source LLC
Chambersburg PA
CBHW060932240326
41458CB00139B/1723